THE ULTIMATE MIND DIET COOKBOOK

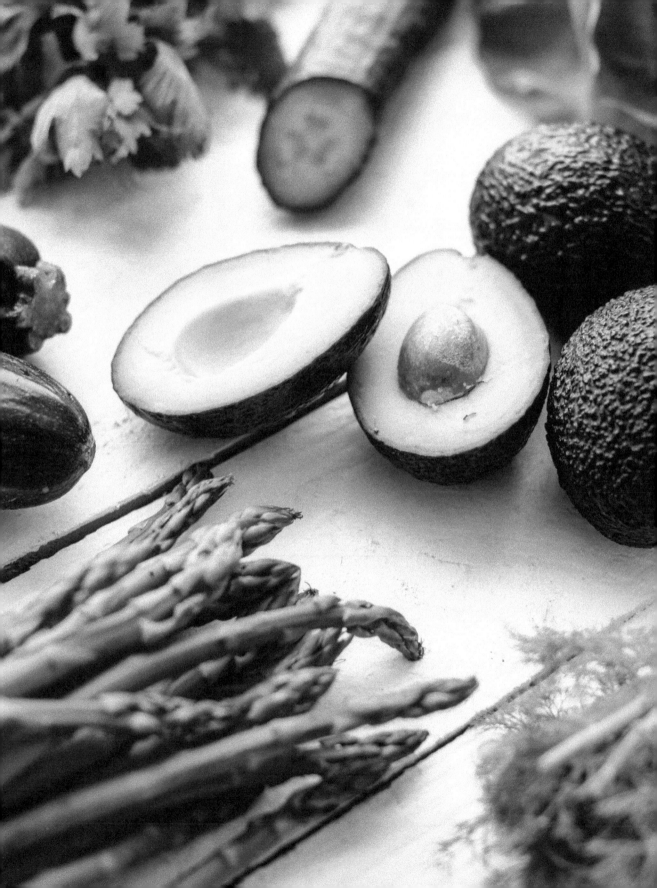

The Ultimate
MIND DIET
COOKBOOK

100 Recipes to Help Prevent Alzheimer's and Dementia

Amanda Foote, RD

ROCKRIDGE
PRESS

For general information on our other products and services or to obtain technical support, please contact our Customer Care Department within the United States at (866) 744-2665, or outside the United States at (510) 253-0500.

Rockridge Press publishes its books in a variety of electronic and print formats. Some content that appears in print may not be available in electronic books, and vice versa.

Interior and Cover Designer: Diana Haas
Art Producer: Michael Hardgrove
Editor: Arturo Conde
Production Editor: Mia Moran
Photography © 2020 Hélène Dujardin. Food styling by Anna Hampton, cover; Stocksy/Ina Peters, p. ii; Darren Muir, pp. vi, 12, 26, 58, 92; Shutterstock, p. viii; Annie Martin, p. x; Shutterstock/Kolpakova Svetlana, p. 40; Stocksy/Nataša Mandić, p. 72; Shutterstock/Timolina, p. 112; Stocksy/Kirsty Begg, p. 132; Elysa Weitala, p. 146
Author photo courtesy of © Brandon Young, Hardstep Design

ISBN: Print 978-1-64611-798-7 | eBook 978-1-64611-799-4
R0

In loving memory of my grandma, Jo.
Dementia never changed the love we shared.
For my grandpa, Dean, whose love, dedication,
and patience were limitless.

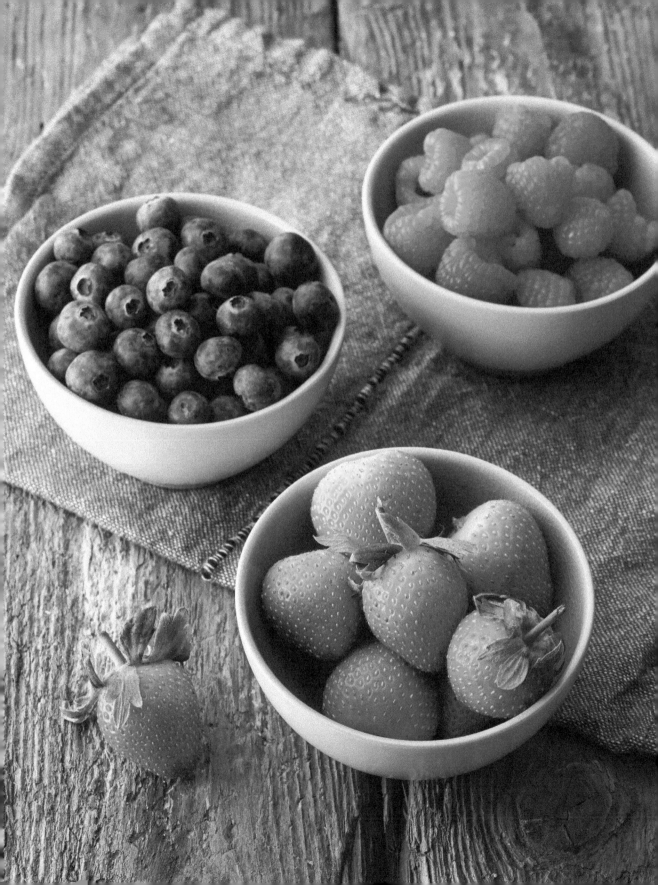

CONTENTS

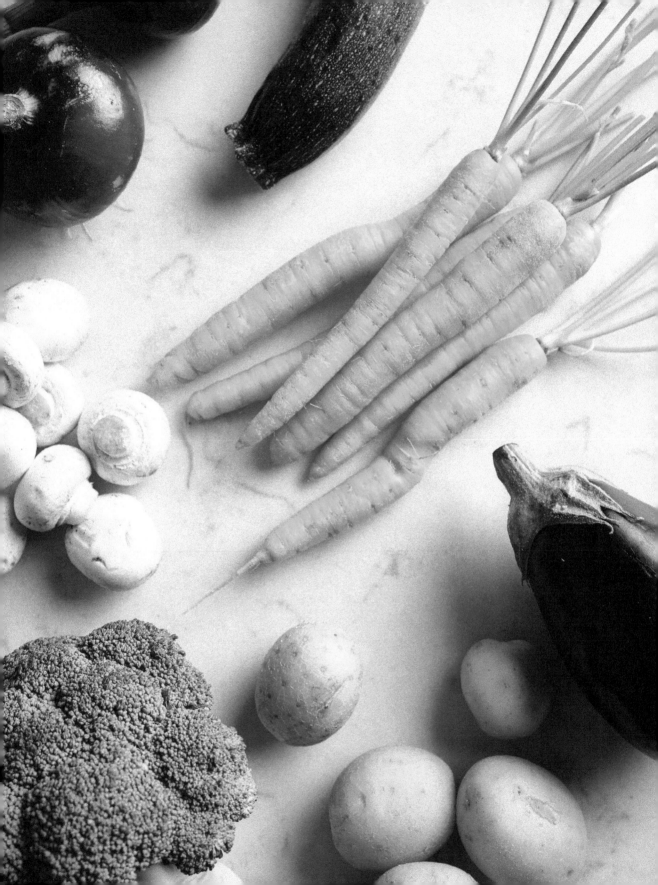

INTRODUCTION

RESEARCH HAS PROVEN time and time again that diets rich in fruits, vegetables, lean protein, and whole grains are beneficial for whole-body health, specifically for the cardiovascular system—and therefore the brain. Based on a combination of two heart-healthy, whole-food-centric eating plans, the Mediterranean and DASH diets, the MIND (Mediterranean-DASH Intervention for Neurodegenerative Delay) diet has been shown to reduce the risk or slow the progression of Alzheimer's disease and dementia.

So how does this diet work? Two major contributing factors that scientists have linked to cognitive decline include inflammation and oxidative stress. To avoid or reduce the severity of these triggers and improve overall health, the MIND diet focuses on antioxidant-rich, plant-based foods and limits (or eliminates) sodium, refined sugar, and saturated/trans fats from daily meals. When combined with an active, healthy lifestyle, this way of eating won't just help you prevent or slow Alzheimer's disease and dementia, it will also leave your whole body feeling stronger and more energized.

This book contains 100 science-backed recipes that will help keep you on track with your MIND diet lifestyle. As you flip through the chapters, you'll find a variety of snacks; soups; salads; grains and legumes; vegan, poultry, and seafood entrées; desserts; and even a recipe for nutrient-packed sangría—all of which are easy to follow, take an hour or less to prepare, and contain ingredients you can find at your local grocery store.

The Ultimate MIND Diet Cookbook is your guide to not only following but also *enjoying* this eating plan. In an effort to help you meet your daily and weekly meal plan goals on the MIND diet, each recipe in this book contains several MIND diet–specific foods to promote brain health and lacks or contains very limited amounts of ingredients that diet researchers recommend avoiding (such as dairy, eggs, red meat, sodium, and refined sugar).

Congratulations for taking this step to improve your life through diet. Food is a powerful tool that can keep your mind and body healthy. And best of all, a healthy, nourishing diet also happens to be full of flavor, comfort, and satisfaction. Welcome to the MIND diet!

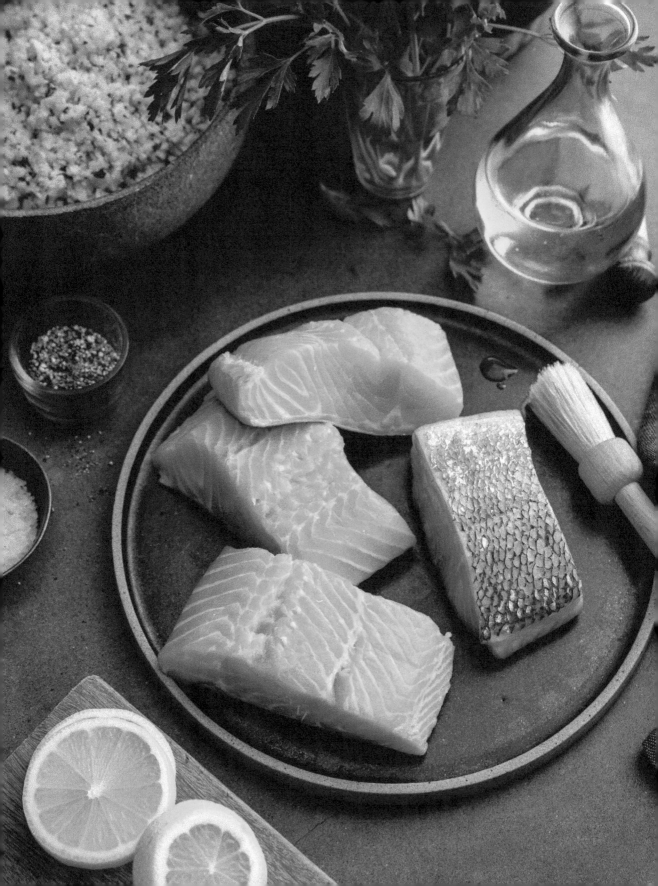

CHAPTER ONE

WHAT YOU SHOULD KNOW ABOUT THE MIND DIET

The idea of using food as a tool for achieving good health traces back to antiquity. The father of medicine, Hippocrates, is famously quoted as saying "Let food be thy medicine, and let medicine be thy food." This is the foundation of the Mediterranean diet and a main reason why people in that region experience less chronic disease. Furthermore, modern medicine strongly supports the idea that a healthy diet can prevent and treat obesity, diabetes, and high blood pressure.

It was long believed that Alzheimer's disease was genetic and dementia was an inevitable result of aging. However, because these two conditions have afflicted the U.S. population at epidemic proportions (Alzheimer's disease is one of the top three causes of death in America, alongside cancer and heart disease), researchers have worked tirelessly to find causes and cures—ultimately discovering that prevention and treatment of cognitive decline can be aided by healthy eating and lifestyle choices.

When followed consistently, the nutrient-rich MIND diet eating plan has been shown to improve cognitive function and reduce the risk and slow the progression of Alzheimer's disease and dementia. The more committed you are to this diet, and the more strictly you follow it, the more likely you will be to see positive results. Here is a closer look at what causes cognitive decline and how the MIND diet can help combat it.

THE SCIENCE

Research on Alzheimer's disease and dementia has found that two key causes of neuron damage are inflammation and oxidative stress, both of which can be prevented and controlled through healthy lifestyle choices such as following a healthy diet, getting sufficient exercise, and avoiding smoking.

OXIDATIVE STRESS is caused by excess free radicals, which come from natural body processes, diet, and environmental pollutants. Free radicals are molecules that are produced when the body breaks down nutrients or is exposed to pollutants like tobacco smoke or radiation. The brain is especially susceptible to oxidative stress because free radicals are created by the same bodily functions that use oxygen, and the brain requires large quantities of oxygen to function. Researchers have found that free radicals may play a role in chronic diseases like heart disease and cancer, and oxidative stress has been directly linked to neurodegenerative disease, including Alzheimer's disease. Oxidative stress can be reduced by eating a diet low in saturated and trans fats and consuming an abundance of antioxidants.

INFLAMMATION is triggered by high blood pressure, high blood sugar, excess body fat, and high blood lipids, and can be controlled by lowering the intake of saturated and trans fats and reducing the use of salt and refined sugar.

Two highly effective diets have been praised for preventing heart disease and high blood pressure, the Mediterranean diet and the DASH diet, and researchers have found that a combination of these heart-healthy eating plans can also help better manage—or even prevent—Alzheimer's disease and dementia.

The Mediterranean diet, based on the traditional eating habits of those who live in the countries bordering the Mediterranean Sea, focuses on vegetables, fruits, herbs, nuts, beans, whole grains, and healthy fats, with lean animal proteins, dairy products, and red wine enjoyed in moderation. In the 1960s, after it was observed that heart disease claimed fewer lives in Mediterranean countries than in other places throughout the world, researchers began to study this cultural way of eating and ultimately concluded that it is indeed effective in lowering rates of cardiovascular disease–related death.

The DASH (Dietary Approaches to Stop Hypertension) diet is based on research funded by the National Institutes of Health, a US government agency devoted to medical research and national health. With a focus on combating hypertension (high blood pressure), this high-fiber, low-fat diet is rich in fruits, vegetables, whole grains, and plant-based oils; allows moderate servings of lean animal proteins, nuts, seeds, and legumes; and limits red meat and sodium.

According to experts, the Mediterranean and DASH diets are both successful in preventing and treating heart disease, high blood pressure, diabetes, inflammation, and oxidative damage, which are all contributing factors to declines in cognitive function. The MIND diet combines specific elements of the Mediterranean and DASH diets—and focuses on specific nutrients known to aid in brain health—with the targeted goal of reducing the risk of or slowing cognitive decline. By combining the inflammation-reducing and oxidative-damage-preventing elements of these two diets, the MIND diet has the power to delay and assist in treating Alzheimer's disease and dementia.

The MIND diet stands for:

M – Mediterranean-DASH

N – Neurodegenerative

I – Intervention for

D – Delay

Here is a breakdown of all three diets' recommendations:

MEDITERRANEAN DIET	DASH DIET	MIND DIET
1. Daily intake of fruits and vegetables, whole grains, and plant oils 2. Weekly intake of lean protein such as poultry, fish and legumes 3. Limited red meat intake 4. Moderate consumption of alcohol and caffeine	1. Daily intake of whole grains, fruits and vegetables, and plant oils 2. No more than once-a-day lean protein such as poultry or fish 3. Several weekly servings of nuts, seeds and legumes 4. Moderate consumption of alcohol and caffeine 5. Limited salt	1. Daily intake of leafy greens, other vegetables, whole grains, and red wine (optional) 2. Multiple weekly servings of nuts, berries, beans/legumes, and poultry 3. At least one weekly serving of seafood 4. Limited intake of saturated fat, trans fat, salt, and refined sugar

Along with other healthy lifestyle choices such as regular exercise and avoiding smoking, the MIND diet is a powerhouse eating plan that—when followed consistently—can help promote a healthy brain for years to come.

PICKING THE BEST FOODS FOR YOUR BRAIN

For the best results, eat a whole-food, mostly plant-based diet, include MIND diet foods in your daily and weekly meals, and limit processed foods and saturated and trans fats. Please note: Though wine is listed as part of the MIND diet, drinking alcohol is a personal choice, and it may not be approved for those with certain health conditions. Talk to your doctor to make sure it is safe for you to consume wine in moderation.

FOODS TO REACH FOR

Though most foods on the MIND diet overlap with those on the DASH and Mediterranean diets, the MIND diet is especially focused on antioxidant-rich foods. Research has shown that antioxidants are responsible for fighting free radicals and thus protecting the body from oxidative stress, which is a leading cause of cognitive decline and neurodegenerative conditions such as Alzheimer's disease and dementia. Here are the key nutrients that help target brain health on the MIND diet, and the foods that contain them:

TYPE OF NUTRIENT	FUNCTION	FOOD SOURCES	
VITAMIN E	An antioxidant that works in the brain to trap free radicals and prevent oxidative damage and protects memory and brain function, helping reduce the risk of developing Alzheimer's disease	• Nuts and seeds • Vegetable oil	
VITAMIN C	An antioxidant that works with vitamin E to prevent oxidative damage	• Broccoli • Brussels sprouts • Cantaloupe • Chiles • Citrus fruits	• Kale • Parsley (fresh) • Strawberries • Sweet peppers • Thyme (fresh)
CAROTENOIDS	Phytonutrients that are responsible for yellow, orange, and red pigments found in fruits and vegetables and that act as antioxidants in the body. Two specific carotenoids—lutein and beta carotene—have been directly linked to preventing dementia.	• Bell peppers • Cantaloupe • Carrots • Dark leafy greens, like kale and spinach	• Oranges • Tomatoes • Watermelon • Wine • Yams
POLYPHENOLS (INCLUDING FLAVONOIDS)	Micronutrients found in fruits, vegetables, and other plants that have antioxidant properties	• Coffee • Dark chocolate • Fruits and vegetables • Herbs and spices	• Lentils and other legumes • Olive oil • Tea • Wine
B VITAMINS	Aid in the prevention of dementia and Alzheimer's disease by helping keep cells healthy and the nervous system functioning properly	• Beans • Leafy green vegetables • Nuts and seeds	• Poultry • Seafood • Whole grains
UNSATURATED FATS	May help reduce the inflammation that causes cognitive aging	• Seafood • Nuts and seeds	• Vegetable oil

FOODS TO CUT BACK ON

Though nothing is completely off limits on the MIND diet, avoiding saturated fats and trans fats is recommended for best results. Diets rich in saturated fat and trans fats can result in increased LDL (bad) cholesterol, which increases the risk of heart disease and can thereby weaken cognitive function. Trans fats can also cause inflammation in the body, which has been linked to an increased risk of heart disease, stroke, diabetes, and neuron damage.

Foods to avoid on the MIND diet because they are high in saturated fat and trans fats include:

- **Dairy products, including butter and cheese**
- **Eggs***
- **Fast food**
- **Fried foods**
- **Margarine**
- **Pastries and sweets**
- **Red meat**

*Eggs are not inherently dangerous to eat. It was long believed that eggs contained too much cholesterol for a healthy diet, but current science shows that most cholesterol is produced naturally in the liver and has less to do with dietary cholesterol intake. The reason caution should be taken with eggs is because of the foods that often accompany eggs that are harmful, such as bacon, sausage, cheese, and pastry. These common accompaniments are high in saturated and trans fats that are unhealthy for the heart and brain. Eggs are a part of a well-rounded diet, but they should always be balanced with whole grains, fruits and vegetables, beans and legumes, nuts and seeds.

SPECIFIC DAILY AND WEEKLY MIND DIET RECOMMENDATIONS

Though the MIND diet includes many of the same foods found in the DASH and Mediterranean diets, its recommendations for *when* and *how much* of those foods you should eat are different. The researchers of the MIND diet have determined that eating specific types of food at specific daily and weekly frequencies helps your body maintain adequate levels of antioxidants, vitamins, minerals, and unsaturated fats, which, in turn, can help prevent cognitive decline such as dementia and Alzheimer's disease. Here are the specific recommendations for daily and weekly intake:

DAILY RECOMMENDATIONS

- 3 servings of whole grains
- 1 salad with leafy greens
- 1 additional serving of vegetables
- 1 glass of red wine (optional)

WEEKLY RECOMMENDATIONS

- Snack on nuts most days
- Eat ½ cup beans or other legumes 3 to 4 times per week
- Have poultry at least 2 times per week
- Eat ½ cup berries at least 2 times per week
- Have fish at least once per week
- Use olive oil for cooking and home-made salad dressings and marinades

BUILDING A KITCHEN FOR YOUR MIND

To be successful on the MIND diet, it is important to stock your kitchen with ingredients that promote healthy cognitive function. Ready to get shopping? Here are the foods you'll be reaching for again and again as you adapt to the MIND diet lifestyle to prevent or slow Alzheimer's disease and dementia.

PANTRY STAPLES

Keeping a well-stocked pantry will make following the MIND diet much easier. Here are some MIND diet pantry staples to always have on hand:

- Black tea bags
- Brown rice
- Canned fruits: pineapple, peaches, pears, mandarin oranges (choose 100% juice varieties with no added sugar, and drain the fruit before eating)
- Canned tomato sauce, tomato paste, diced or crushed tomatoes (choose no-salt-added varieties)
- Canned vegetables: corn, green beans, peas, etc. (choose no-salt-added varieties)
- Coffee
- Corn tortillas
- Dark chocolate
- Dried herbs and spices: garlic powder, onion powder, black pepper, chili pepper, cayenne pepper, oregano, parsley, Italian seasoning, basil, turmeric, ginger, bay leaves, cinnamon, cumin, curry powder, dill, paprika, rosemary, thyme, vanilla extract
- Dried lentils: red, yellow, brown, green

- Dried or canned beans: black, pinto, kidney, white, cannellini, navy, chickpeas, black-eyed peas, soybeans (if canned, choose no-salt-added varieties)
- Dried split peas
- Green tea bags
- Light tuna canned in water
- Low-sodium chicken stock
- Low-sodium vegetable stock
- Old-fashioned rolled oats
- Olive oil
- Quinoa
- Red wine (optional)
- Unsalted nuts
- Unsalted seeds
- Whole-grain bread
- Whole-grain pasta

FRESH PRODUCE

A refrigerator full of fresh produce is another powerful tool that will help you stay on track and reap the most benefits from the MIND diet. Rotate your stock of these vitamin- and mineral-rich ingredients depending on the meals you are planning each week.

VEGETABLES

- Asparagus
- Bell peppers
- Broccoli
- Cabbage
- Carrots
- Cauliflower
- Celery
- Chiles
- Garlic
- Kale
- Leafy greens
- Mixed spring greens
- Mushrooms
- Onions
- Romaine lettuce
- Spinach
- Squash
- Sweet peppers
- Tomatoes
- Yams/sweet potatoes

FRUITS

- Blueberries
- Lemons
- Limes
- Raspberries
- Strawberries

LEAN PROTEIN

Lean protein is a key component of the MIND diet. Buy it fresh every week depending on the meals you plan to make, or save some money by buying your favorite lean protein options in bulk and stocking them in the freezer (chicken, turkey, and fish can be frozen for up to 6 months). Examples of MIND diet–approved lean proteins include:

- Boneless, skinless chicken breast
- Ground turkey
- Salmon
- Tofu
- Turkey breast or cutlets

ABOUT THE RECIPES

All the recipes and ingredients in this cookbook are MIND diet approved and have been carefully selected to illustrate how easy—and delicious—it can be to adapt to an eating plan that can prevent or slow the progression of Alzheimer's disease and dementia. Not only will you enjoy a rainbow of leafy salads and nutrient-packed vegetable dishes, but you'll also find satisfying breakfasts to start the day off right, new ways to prepare lean proteins like chicken and fish, cozy soups and stews, and even desserts and drinks (alcohol optional). Armed with the 100 recipes in the chapters that follow, you'll be able to craft weekly MIND diet menus that will nourish your body and brain without skimping on flavor.

As a reminder, the MIND diet excludes dairy, eggs, red meat, trans fats, and saturated fats, and allows for only minimal amounts of salt and sugar. The recipes in this book reflect these restrictions and feature foods that are specifically beneficial to brain health and the prevention or slowing of Alzheimer's disease and dementia. You'll find the MIND diet superfoods highlighted in the ingredient list of each recipe, so you can learn what foods fit into your diet to easily meet your meal plan requirements.

For your convenience, the recipes also contain handy tips for making nutritious MIND diet meals:

- COOKING TIPS: Helpful insights to make the dish easier to prepare, cook, or clean up.

- **INGREDIENT TIPS:** Provide more information about specific ingredients, such as how to select produce, best practices for preparation, and nutrition facts.

- **SUBSTITUTION TIPS:** Helpful if you have food allergies or intolerances or would like to make flavor changes to the recipe.

- **VARIATION TIPS:** Suggestions for adding or changing ingredients to mix things up a little or try something new with the recipe.

At the beginning of most of the recipes, you will find at least one of the following labels, which will help you choose dishes that fit within your time constraints, dietary restrictions, and preferences:

- **30 MINUTES:** Requires less than 30 minutes to prepare, from start to finish.

- **CONTAINS NUTS OR SEEDS:** Not suitable for people who are allergic to nuts or seeds. In these recipes, you can simply omit the nuts and still cook a delicious dish.

- **GLUTEN-FREE:** Not suitable for people who have celiac disease or gluten sensitivity. Any recipe that contains gluten can be made with a gluten-free alternative such as rice pasta, quinoa, or gluten-free flour. Always check packaging for gluten-free labeling to ensure that foods were prepared in a totally gluten-free facility.

- **ONE-POT:** Can be prepared in one pot, allowing flavors to marry thoroughly with the added benefit of fewer dirty dishes.

- **SLOW COOKER:** Requires more time than other recipes, as the ingredients need to cook for several hours. Recipes with this label will need to be started well in advance of mealtime.

- **VEGAN:** Is completely plant based, containing no meat, poultry, seafood, dairy, honey, or eggs.

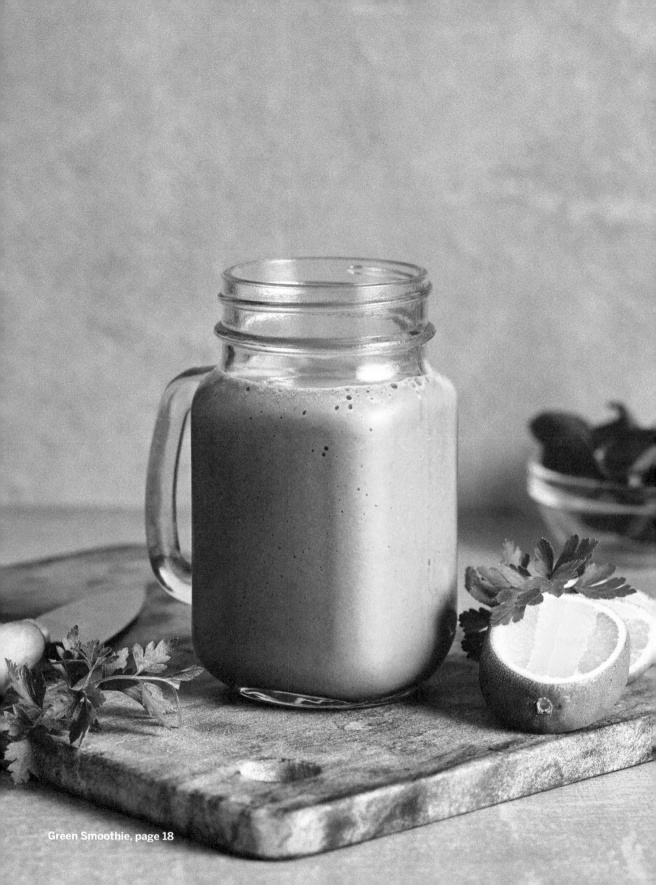

Green Smoothie, page 18

BREAKFAST AND SMOOTHIES

Adequate nutrient intake, regardless of the time of day, is vital to good health and prevention of chronic disease such as Alzheimer's disease and dementia. However, starting the day with a healthy meal is especially helpful, as it provides great momentum to make healthy choices through the afternoon and evening. Breakfast is the first opportunity of every day to fuel your body with vitamins, minerals, antioxidants, and energy, and people who take the time to eat a nutritious breakfast tend to be more alert and experience better concentration, memory, and cognitive function than those who skip this meal.

When you discover how easy it is to whip up the smoothies and other recipes in this chapter, you'll never be tempted to pass on the first meal of the day again. Most of these MIND diet breakfast recipes are ready in 5 minutes, with some exceptions taking up to 40 minutes to prepare—perfect for lazy weekend mornings. And, of course, every recipe in this chapter was created based on strong MIND diet nutrients. It's never been easier to start the day off right!

MIND DIET SUPERHEROES: BERRIES

Berries help prevent and reduce symptoms from many chronic diseases. They are a particularly good source of antioxidants, which are vitally important to fight the free radicals that cause oxidative stress—a known catalyst for neuron damage associated with Alzheimer's disease and dementia. It is recommended to eat ½ cup of berries at least twice per week on the MIND diet.

You will find 11 recipes in this book that feature berries, from breakfasts and snacks to entrées and desserts. Enjoy the Spelt Pancakes with Berry Compote (page 24) on a relaxing Saturday morning. Blend up a Mixed Berry Smoothie (page 19) or Grains and Berries Smoothie Bowl (page 17) for a quick breakfast before you run out the door. Pack a snack bag of Sweet Nut Mix (page 38) for your afternoon cravings. Toss together a Strawberry-Spinach Salad (page 54) or Cranberry-Chicken Salad (page 46) for your lunch, and Cranberry-Walnut Broccoli Slaw (page 47) or Turkey-Cranberry Rice (page 127) for dinner. Relax on the porch with a glass of alcoholic or nonalcoholic Sangría (page 144) or a bowl of Berry Oat Crisp (page 136) with Berry "Nice Cream" (page 135) to give a sweet finish to your day.

AVOCADO-OATMEAL BREAKFAST BARS

CONTAINS NUTS, GLUTEN-FREE
SERVES 4 / PREP TIME: 10 MINUTES / COOK TIME: 30 MINUTES

Eggs can be replaced one for one with mashed banana, and butter can be replaced with avocado, a healthy source of plant-based fat. These breakfast bars have a chewy, dense texture and will keep you full for hours.

1 ripe banana, mashed

1 small ripe avocado, pitted, peeled, and mashed

2 tablespoons peanut butter

2 tablespoons honey

2 cups old-fashioned rolled oats

2 tablespoons water

1 teaspoon vanilla extract

¼ cup vegan dark chocolate chips or chunks (optional)

1. Preheat the oven to 350°F.

2. In a mixing bowl, combine all the ingredients.

3. In a parchment paper–lined 9-by-9-inch pan, press the mixture into an even layer.

4. Bake for 30 minutes, until the edges begin to brown and crisp.

5. Let cool for 10 minutes.

6. Cut into squares or rectangles and serve.

SUBSTITUTION TIP: Any nut butter will work in this recipe if you want some variety from peanut butter, though peanut butter and banana and chocolate are a wonderful marriage of flavors. You could easily add chopped nuts to this recipe for some added crunch and extra protein and fiber.

PER SERVING: Calories: 313; Total fat: 12g; Protein: 8g; Carbohydrates: 47g; Fiber: 8g; Sugar: 15g; Sodium: 40mg

CITRUS SMOOTHIE

GLUTEN-FREE, ONE-POT, 30 MINUTES, VEGAN
SERVES 2 TO 4 / PREP TIME: 10 MINUTES

Citrus fruits are a friendly staple in many kitchens, and while they are familiar and delicious, they are also excellent sources of vitamins and minerals. While most think of citrus fruits for vitamin C, they are also rich in antioxidants, B vitamins, and fiber, and they reduce inflammation. This recipe features grapefruit and orange but would work with lemons or limes as well.

2 oranges, peeled and sectioned, frozen

1 red grapefruit, peeled and sectioned, frozen

1 red beet, peeled and diced

1 teaspoon ground turmeric

1 teaspoon ground ginger

½ cup ice cubes

½ cup unsweetened plain nondairy milk

1. In a blender, blend all the ingredients on high, or on the smoothie setting for 30 to 60 seconds.

2. Add additional liquid as desired and reblend.

3. Serve chilled.

COOKING TIP: For a thicker smoothie for a smoothie bowl, add liquid ¼ cup at a time until the desired consistency is reached.

PER SERVING: Calories: 139; Total fat: 1g; Protein: 3g; Carbohydrates: 33g; Fiber: 7g; Sugar: 15g; Sodium: 76mg

GRAINS AND BERRIES SMOOTHIE BOWL

CONTAINS SEEDS, 30 MINUTES, VEGAN
SERVES 2 TO 4 / PREP TIME: 5 MINUTES

This recipe gives your artistic abilities a chance to shine. Decorating your smoothie bowl with toppings is the best part, adding colors, textures, and flavors to an already tasty breakfast.

FOR THE SMOOTHIE

1 cup blueberries, frozen

1 cup raspberries, frozen

2 bananas, sliced and frozen

¼ cup unsweetened plain or vanilla nondairy milk

FOR THE TOPPINGS

½ cup sliced strawberries

½ cup Grape-Nuts cereal

1 tablespoon shaved coconut

1 teaspoon flaxseed

1. In a blender, blend the blueberries, raspberries, bananas, and nondairy milk on high, or on the smoothie setting for 30 to 60 seconds.

2. Pour the smoothie into a bowl.

3. Decorate with the toppings and serve.

COOKING TIP: Enjoying a smoothie bowl is a lot like enjoying sorbet; you can eat the smoothie with a spoon. If needed, add additional liquid 1 tablespoon at a time until the desired consistency is reached.

VARIATION TIP: A spoonful of nut butter is a great addition to this smoothie bowl. You can also replace the flaxseed with chia seeds or hemp seeds.

PER SERVING: Calories: 324; Total fat: 4g; Protein: 7g; Carbohydrates: 71g; Fiber: 15g; Sugar: 29g; Sodium: 170mg

GREEN SMOOTHIE

CONTAINS SEEDS, GLUTEN-FREE, ONE-POT, 30 MINUTES, VEGAN
SERVES 2 TO 4 / PREP TIME: 10 MINUTES

Green smoothies have gained a lot of attention in the media and with celebrities. While they might seem trendy, they are a wonderful choice on the MIND diet. Rich in vitamins, minerals, antioxidants, and fiber, green smoothies are an easy and delicious way to add a serving of leafy green vegetables to your diet.

2 bananas, sliced and frozen

2 cups fresh spinach, packed

1 cup fresh pineapple chunks

1 tablespoon flaxseed

1 cup ice

1 cup water

1. In a blender, blend all the ingredients on high until smooth, or on the smoothie setting for 30 to 60 seconds. For a thinner smoothie, add ½ cup more water 1 tablespoon at a time until the desired consistency is reached.

2. Serve chilled.

INGREDIENT TIP: You can use canned pineapple in this recipe. Simply purchase pineapple in 100 percent fruit juice and drain the juice before adding to the blender.

PER SERVING: Calories: 168; Total fat: 2g; Protein: 3g; Carbohydrates: 39g; Fiber: 6g; Sugar: 22g; Sodium: 27mg

MIXED BERRY SMOOTHIE

GLUTEN-FREE, ONE-POT, 30 MINUTES, VEGAN
SERVES 2 TO 4 / PREP TIME: 5 MINUTES

Cinnamon sweetens and spices this smoothie, and nutmeg provides a spiciness and nuttiness. Cinnamon and nutmeg are both wonder spices that are packed with antioxidants and help reduce inflammation. Combined with the berries in this recipe, this smoothie is an antioxidant powerhouse.

1 cup blueberries, frozen

1 cup raspberries, frozen

1 cup blackberries, frozen

1 teaspoon ground cinnamon

1 teaspoon ground nutmeg

2 cups unsweetened plain or vanilla nondairy milk

1. In a blender, blend all the ingredients on high until smooth, or on the smoothie setting for 30 to 60 seconds.

2. Add additional liquid as needed and reblend.

3. Serve chilled.

SUBSTITUTION TIP: Any blend of berries would work in this recipe. Strawberries, cranberries, boysenberries, gooseberries, or açai berries would all pack a nutrient-dense tangy punch to this smoothie.

COOKING TIP: For a thicker smoothie for a smoothie bowl, add liquid ¼ cup at a time until the desired consistency is reached.

PER SERVING: Calories: 162; Total fat: 4g; Protein: 3g; Carbohydrates: 32g; Fiber: 12g; Sugar: 18g; Sodium: 172mg

MOCHA-BANANA SMOOTHIE

GLUTEN-FREE, ONE-POT, 30 MINUTES, VEGAN
SERVES 2 TO 4 / PREP TIME: 5 MINUTES

Carrots are a surprising addition to this smoothie. They are sweet and full of antioxidants, vitamins, and minerals, and you won't even notice them behind the robust chocolate and coffee flavors.

4 bananas, sliced and frozen

2 carrots, sliced and frozen

2 tablespoons unsweetened cocoa powder

2 cups brewed coffee, chilled

1. In a blender, blend all the ingredients on high, or on the smoothie setting for 30 to 60 seconds.

2. Add additional liquid as needed and reblend for a thinner smoothie or add a few ice cubes and reblend for a thicker smoothie.

3. Serve chilled.

COOKING TIP: Freezing leftover carrot pieces is a great way to reduce food waste and have them ready in the freezer for this recipe.

VARIATION TIP: Add ½ teaspoon cayenne pepper for a Mexican hot chocolate vibe, or fresh mint leaves for a mint chocolate treat.

PER SERVING: Calories: 250; Total fat: 2g; Protein: 5g; Carbohydrates: 63g; Fiber: 10g; Sugar: 32g; Sodium: 51mg

PEANUT BUTTER AND CHOCOLATE SMOOTHIE

CONTAINS NUTS, GLUTEN-FREE, ONE-POT, 30 MINUTES, VEGAN

SERVES 4 / PREP TIME: 5 MINUTES

Peanuts are a nutrient powerhouse, rich in fiber, vitamins, minerals, protein, and healthy fat. They pack the same health benefits as more expensive nuts and are readily accessible and more affordable.

4 bananas, sliced and frozen

½ cup creamy peanut butter

1 tablespoon unsweetened cocoa powder

2 cups unsweetened plain or vanilla nondairy milk

1. In a blender, blend all the ingredients on high until smooth, or on the smoothie setting for 30 to 60 seconds.

2. Add additional liquid as needed and reblend for a thinner smoothie or add a few ice cubes and reblend for a thicker smoothie.

3. Serve chilled.

COOKING TIP: Freezing bananas before they get too ripe is a perfect way to have frozen bananas ready for smoothies. Simply dice the ripe bananas and freeze in a freezer-safe container or bag.

PER SERVING: Calories: 312, Total fat: 18g; Carbohydrates: 35g; Fiber: 6g; Sugars: 18g, Protein: 10g; Sodium: 234mg

SCRAMBLED TOFU

GLUTEN-FREE, ONE-POT, VEGAN
SERVES 4 / PREP TIME: 30 MINUTES / COOK TIME: 5 MINUTES

Tofu is soybean curd that is pressed into a block and is an excellent source of vegetable-based protein and strong antioxidants. A blank canvas, tofu perfectly takes on marinades and seasonings.

14 ounces extra-firm tofu

1 teaspoon olive oil

1 teaspoon ground turmeric

¼ teaspoon onion powder

¼ teaspoon garlic powder

1 cup grape or cherry tomatoes, quartered

1. Line a plate with several paper towels. Remove the tofu block from the package and place on the paper towels.

2. Add additional paper towels on top of the tofu block and place a cutting board on top of the paper towels.

3. Weigh the cutting board down with a heavy book, a pot, or several cans.

4. Leave the tofu to drain for at least 30 minutes.

5. In a large sauté pan or skillet, heat the olive oil on medium heat and add the block of tofu.

6. Mash the tofu into small curds with a potato masher.

7. Stir in the turmeric, onion powder, garlic powder, and tomatoes and sauté together for 5 minutes. Serve.

COOKING TIP: Pressing your tofu takes time but is worth the effort. Watery tofu cooks down to be overly soft, whereas pressed tofu retains its firmness and, without holding water, can absorb more flavor from your seasonings of choice.

PER SERVING: Calories: 114; Total fat: 6g; Protein: 11g; Carbohydrates: 6g; Fiber: 2g; Sugar: 1g; Sodium: 33mg

VEGETABLE-AVOCADO TOAST

ONE-POT, 30 MINUTES, VEGAN
SERVES 4 / PREP TIME: 5 MINUTES / COOK TIME: 5 MINUTES

Avocados are a wonderful fruit that can serve as a creamy butter or mayonnaise substitute. They are a good source of omega-3 fatty acids, antioxidants, and numerous vitamins and minerals. Avocados are also a good source of fiber, and while they are full of fat, it is the kind of fat that benefits your health.

1 large avocado

1 beet, peeled

4 pieces of whole-grain bread

1 cup fresh arugula

2 tablespoons olive oil

1 teaspoon cracked black pepper

1. Remove the pit, peel the avocado, and cut into 4 portions; set aside.

2. Shave the beet on a box grater; set aside.

3. Toast the bread to your liking.

4. Top the toast with the avocado, arugula, and shaved beets.

5. Drizzle the toast with olive oil, sprinkle with cracked pepper, and serve.

SUBSTITUTION TIP: Any vegetables would be delicious on avocado toast. You could substitute any leafy green, tomato, bell pepper, shaved carrots, or even add black beans and salsa.

PER SERVING: Calories: 272; Total fat: 16g; Protein: 7g; Carbohydrates: 29g; Fiber: 9g; Sugar: 7g; Sodium: 201mg

SPELT PANCAKES WITH BERRY COMPOTE

CONTAINS SEEDS, 30 MINUTES, VEGAN

SERVES 4 / PREP TIME: 10 MINUTES / COOK TIME: 20 MINUTES

These dairy-free pancakes feature a flax "egg," which is an egg substitute made from warm water and ground flaxseed. The flax egg allows the ingredients to stretch and rise just like an egg would, but with the added benefit of omega-3 fatty acids, antioxidants, and fiber.

FOR THE COMPOTE

1 cup fresh or frozen berries, any variety

1 tablespoon 100% fruit juice, any variety

FOR THE FLAX EGG

1 tablespoon ground flaxseed

2½ tablespoons warm water

FOR THE PANCAKES

1 cup spelt flour

1 tablespoon baking powder

1 cup unsweetened vanilla nondairy milk

1 tablespoon lemon juice

1 teaspoon agave syrup

1. For the compote, in a small pot, combine the berries and fruit juice.

2. Bring to a boil, cover, and reduce heat to medium.

3. Cook the compote for 5 to 10 minutes, stirring frequently. The mixture will reduce by half. Set aside.

4. While the compote is cooking, in a small bowl, combine the flaxseed and warm water. Set aside to gel together.

5. In a medium bowl, whisk together the spelt flour and the baking powder for the pancakes.

6. Add the nondairy milk, lemon juice, agave syrup, and flax egg, and whisk into the dry ingredients until all the ingredients are well incorporated.

7. Preheat a skillet or griddle on medium heat.

8. Add ¼ cup of the batter at a time to the skillet or griddle to make small pancakes.

9. Leave the batter alone for about 3 minutes and watch for small bubbles to start appearing on top of the pancakes.

10. Flip the pancakes gently and allow to cook on the second side for another 3 minutes.

11. Serve each pancake topped with the berry compote.

SUBSTITUTION TIP: Chia seeds can also be used to make a chia "egg" in the same water-to-seed ratio.

VARIATION TIP: This berry compote is a simple recipe that you can easily add flavors to. Cinnamon, ginger, or lemon zest will pleasantly change the flavor of your compote, which is a perfect substitute for syrup on these spelt pancakes.

PER SERVING: Calories: 166; Total fat: 2g; Protein: 5g; Carbohydrates: 31g; Fiber: 6g; Sugar: 6g; Sodium: 412mg

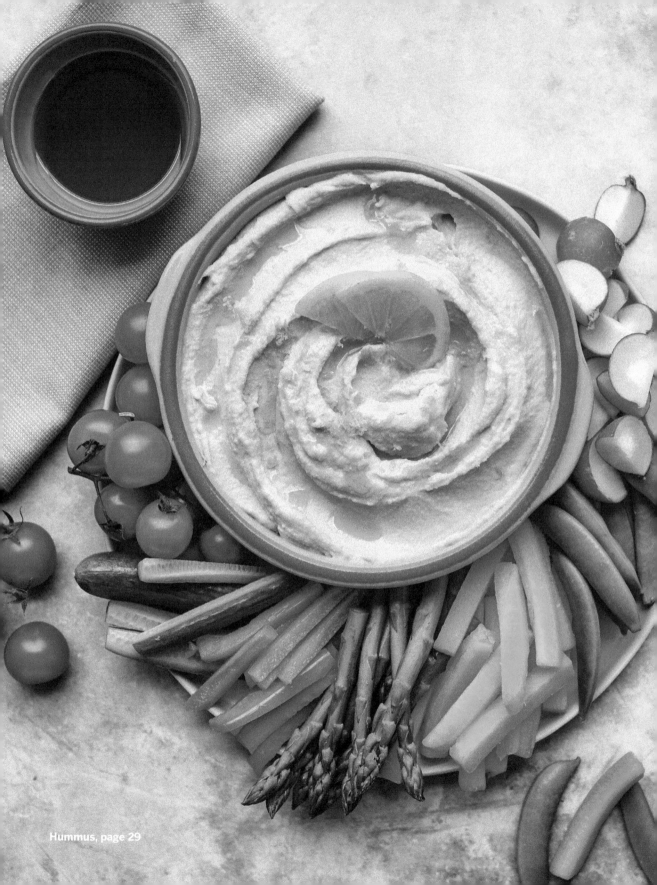

Hummus, page 29

CHAPTER THREE

SNACKS

For many of us, when we crave a snack, we reach for something premade in a wrapper. A salty or crunchy craving may have you reaching for a bag of chips, and a sweet craving may have you reaching for one (or five) bite-size candy bars. Snacking does not have to mean potato chips with French onion dip from a jar, or an entire row of cookies, and ignoring hunger isn't the answer, either, since that will only guarantee overeating later in the day. The MIND diet is bountiful in recommended nutrients, and snack time is an opportunity to vary your intake and satisfy cravings at the same time. It is recommended to consume 3 servings of whole grains per day, to eat ½ cup beans 3 to 4 times per week, and to snack on nuts most days. The snacks in this chapter are made with a variety of whole grains, beans, and nuts, featuring many different flavor combinations to keep your palate excited.

SNACK FACTS

Various studies have shown that the average American eats at least two snacks per day, accounting for one-quarter of their daily caloric intake, and according to a 2011 report by the USDA Food Surveys Research Group, the percentage of adults snacking went up from 59 percent in the 1970s to 90 percent in the early 2000s. Although it is often thought of as an unhealthy habit, when you make good food choices, snacking can actually be a great way to stay satisfied and energized between meals and include more MIND-friendly nutrients in your diet.

The MIND diet snack recipes in this chapter can satisfy cravings, boost energy, and nourish your body. Get a long-lasting energy boost and fullness from the protein and healthy fats in the nut mixes (pages 33, 36, 37, and 38), Hummus (page 29), and Roasted Chickpeas (page 35). Satisfy your need for crunch with the Whole-Grain Snack Mix (page 39) and the popcorn mixes (pages 33 and 34). Easily incorporate vegetables into your snack routine with Kale Chips (page 32) or Corn Chips with Guacamole and Salsa (page 30). When you choose the right foods, snacking can be a healthy and regular element of your MIND diet eating plan.

HUMMUS

CONTAINS SEEDS, GLUTEN-FREE, 30 MINUTES, VEGAN
SERVES 4 / PREP TIME: 10 MINUTES / COOK TIME: 20 MINUTES

Chickpeas are a plant-based protein powerhouse. Rich in fiber, manganese, copper, and folate, these marble-size beans are a versatile pantry staple. Both tahini (sesame seed butter) and olive oil are rich in antioxidants with anti-inflammatory properties. Hummus can be served with pita chips or crackers, as a vegetable dip, and in wraps and sandwiches.

1 (15-ounce) can chickpeas, drained and rinsed

2 cups water

¼ teaspoon baking soda

2 tablespoons lemon juice

1 teaspoon minced garlic

2 tablespoons ice-cold water

⅓ cup tahini

1 tablespoon olive oil

1. In a medium saucepan, cover the chickpeas with water, and add the baking soda.

2. Boil the chickpeas for 20 minutes, until the skins are falling off.

3. Drain and rinse the chickpeas.

4. In a blender or food processor, combine the chickpeas with the lemon juice, minced garlic, ice-cold water, and tahini and blend until creamy and smooth, 2 to 3 minutes.

5. Serve in a bowl with the olive oil drizzled on top.

VARIATION TIP: Hummus can be flavored just about any way you like. Add roasted red peppers for a smoky-flavored hummus, or avocado for a guacamole-like dip with the added benefit of protein. Add pumpkin purée or sweet potato with cumin, chili powder, and a chipotle pepper for a spicy-sweet hummus. You can even make dessert hummus by omitting the garlic and lemon juice and adding cocoa powder, vanilla extract, and dark chocolate chips, and serve with fruit.

SUBSTITUTION TIP: Sunflower butter and almond butter are suitable alternatives to tahini for anyone allergic to sesame, or if you do not have tahini on hand. If chickpeas are not your favorite, you can easily replace them with black beans or white beans and achieve a similar result.

PER SERVING: Calories: 255; Total fat: 15g; Protein: 9g; Carbohydrates: 24g; Fiber: 7g; Sugar: <1g; Sodium: 103mg

CORN CHIPS WITH GUACAMOLE AND SALSA

GLUTEN-FREE, 30 MINUTES, VEGAN

SERVES 4 / PREP TIME: 15 MINUTES / COOK TIME: 10 MINUTES

This snack is the best of all worlds: whole grains, fruits, vegetables, fiber, healthy fat, vitamins, minerals, and antioxidants. Corn is a whole grain, and, in this preparation, has no added salt or fat. Masa for corn tortillas is made of ground corn and water. Avocados are rich in omega-3 fatty acids, and tomatoes are rich in antioxidants. This guacamole and salsa can be spiced up or toned down to your liking.

16 corn tortillas

2 tablespoons olive oil

1 tablespoon smoked paprika

2 medium avocados, pitted, peeled, and diced

1 medium white onion, finely diced, divided

1 jalapeño, finely diced, divided

3 large hothouse tomatoes, diced, divided

1 tablespoon minced garlic

1 lime, halved

1. Preheat the oven to 350°F.

2. While the oven is preheating, brush the corn tortillas with olive oil and sprinkle evenly with smoked paprika.

3. Cut the seasoned tortillas into quarters.

4. On a parchment paper–lined baking sheet, arrange the tortilla pieces in a single layer, or as close to a single layer as your pan size will allow.

5. Bake the tortilla pieces for 10 minutes, until they begin to brown. The chips may feel soft but will crisp further as they cool.

6. While the chips are cooking, begin preparing the guacamole and salsa. In a medium bowl, mash the avocados until mostly smooth.

7. Add half of the diced onion, half of the diced jalapeño, and one-third of the diced tomato. Set the guacamole aside.

8. In a blender or food processor, combine the remaining diced onion, jalapeño, and tomato, the minced garlic, and the juice from one half of the lime. Blend to the desired consistency. Pour the salsa into a bowl and set aside.

9. When the chips are done baking, squeeze the juice from the remaining lime half over the chips. Allow to cool for 10 minutes.

10. Serve together as a delicious light snack.

INGREDIENT TIP: When shopping for corn tortillas, touch is a must to choose a good package. Lightly bend the package to see if the tortillas are fresh. If the tortillas appear to be separate and do not stick together, and are pliable, they are fresh. Corn tortillas made from small or family-run tortillerias tend to be fresher than tortillas that are mass-produced.

PER SERVING: Calories: 484; Total fat: 24g; Protein: 10g; Carbohydrates: 66g; Fiber: 16g; Sugar: 7g; Sodium: 68mg

KALE CHIPS

GLUTEN-FREE, ONE-POT, 30 MINUTES, VEGAN
SERVES 4 / PREP TIME: 10 MINUTES / COOK TIME: 20 MINUTES

Kale chips are a simple, healthy alternative to crunchy, salty snacks such as potato chips and crackers. Some simple tips will ensure you make delicious kale chips every time. The leaves will shrink as they bake, so keep them larger "chip" size. Bake in a single layer to achieve maximum crisp. Kale chips are best when eaten fresh, before moisture can cause them to go limp.

1 bunch fresh kale, thoroughly rinsed and dried

1 tablespoon olive oil

¼ teaspoon freshly ground black pepper

1. Preheat the oven to 225°F.

2. Remove the kale leaves from the woody stems and cut into large "chip" sizes.

3. Combine the kale, olive oil, and black pepper in a gallon zip-top bag.

4. Seal and shake vigorously to ensure the oil and pepper reach every nook and cranny of the kale leaves.

5. Place on a baking sheet in a single layer and bake for 10 minutes.

6. Flip the kale chips and bake for another 10 minutes. Watch the kale chips and remove before they begin to burn.

7. Serve while warm.

VARIATION TIP: Kale is a blank canvas for flavorings, so you can go wild with any variation you think sounds delicious. Try lemon juice and pepper, ginger and cayenne pepper, or garlic powder and dill. The combinations are endless.

PER SERVING: Calories: 58; Total fat: 4g; Protein: 2g; Carbohydrates: 6g; Fiber: 2g; Sugar: 1g; Sodium: 23mg

POPCORN NUT MIX

CONTAINS NUTS, GLUTEN-FREE, ONE-POT, 30 MINUTES, VEGAN
SERVES 4 / PREP TIME: 5 MINUTES / COOK TIME: 5 MINUTES

Popcorn is a whole-grain, low-calorie, high-fiber, perfect snack. High in manganese, magnesium, phosphorus, and zinc, popcorn is a vitamin- and mineral-rich food welcomed on the MIND diet. Popcorn is also high in polyphenol antioxidants, helping protect the body from free radicals. Another wonderful thing about popcorn is that a serving is 4 to 5 cups!

2 tablespoons olive oil

½ cup popcorn kernels

1 cup almonds

1 tablespoon dried rosemary

¼ teaspoon salt

¼ teaspoon garlic powder

1. In a large stockpot, heat the olive oil on medium heat until shimmering.

2. Add the popcorn kernels and cover the stockpot.

3. The kernels will pop for 4 to 5 minutes. Listen closely. When the popping slows to only every few seconds, your popcorn is done.

4. Toss the popcorn and nuts together with the seasonings and serve.

COOKING TIP: Place 2 popcorn kernels in the bottom of the stockpot while it heats up. When those 2 kernels have popped, add the remaining kernels. This will ensure the oil is hot enough to evenly pop all the kernels.

PER SERVING: Calories: 367; Total fat: 26g; Protein: 10g; Carbohydrates: 28g; Fiber: 10g; Sugar: 2g; Sodium: 146mg

POPCORN WITH FLAVOR MIX-INS

GLUTEN-FREE, ONE-POT, 30 MINUTES, VEGAN

SERVES 4 / PREP TIME: 5 MINUTES / COOK TIME: 5 MINUTES

Popcorn isn't just for the movies anymore! Gone are the days of butter-loaded, salt-laden popcorn in front of a screen. Here are the days of snacking on popcorn as a whole-grain, healthy MIND diet staple. Loaded with the seasonings of your choice, this snack will never grow old.

FOR THE POPCORN

2 tablespoons olive oil

½ cup popcorn kernels

SALSA EN POLVO MIX-IN

1 tablespoon chili powder

1 tablespoon lime zest

¼ teaspoon salt

RANCH MIX-IN

½ teaspoon dried dill weed

½ teaspoon dried chives

½ teaspoon garlic powder

½ teaspoon onion powder

HOT COCOA MIX-IN

1 tablespoon unsweetened cocoa powder

1 teaspoon sugar

½ teaspoon ground cinnamon

CHURRO MIX-IN

1 tablespoon ground cinnamon

1 teaspoon sugar

1. In a large stockpot, heat the olive oil on medium heat until shimmering.

2. Add the popcorn kernels and cover the stockpot.

3. The kernels will pop for 4 to 5 minutes. Listen closely. When the popping slows to only every few seconds, your popcorn is done.

4. While hot, toss the popcorn in your choice of seasonings and serve.

COOKING TIP: Place 2 popcorn kernels in the bottom of the stockpot while it heats up. When those 2 kernels have popped, add the remaining kernels. This will ensure the oil is hot enough to evenly pop all the kernels.

SALSA: Per serving: Calories: 167; Total fat: 8g; Protein: 2g; Carbohydrates: 21g; Fiber: 6g; Sugar: <1g; Sodium: 164mg

RANCH: Per serving: Calories: 163; Total fat: 8g; Protein: 2g; Carbohydrates: 21g; Fiber: 5g; Sugar: 0g; Sodium: 1mg

COCOA: Per serving: Calories: 168; Total fat: 8g; Protein: 2g; Carbohydrates: 22g; Fiber: 6g; Sugar: 1g; Sodium: <1mg

CHURRO: Per serving: Calories: 168; Total fat: 8g; Protein: 2g; Carbohydrates: 22g; Fiber: 6g; Sugar: 1g; Sodium: <1mg

ROASTED CHICKPEAS

GLUTEN-FREE, VEGAN

SERVES 4 / PREP TIME: 5 MINUTES / COOK TIME: 45 MINUTES

Rich in protein, roasted chickpeas make a perfect snack. Make sure to dry the chickpeas well, and thoroughly coated with olive oil to reach maximum crunchiness. These roasted chickpeas work deliciously as a crouton substitute on a salad or make a crunchy soup topping.

1 (15-ounce) can chickpeas, drained, rinsed, and blotted dry

1 tablespoon olive oil

¼ teaspoon chili powder

¼ teaspoon garlic powder

1. Preheat the oven to 450°F.

2. In a large bowl, toss the chickpeas in the olive oil.

3. On a parchment paper–lined baking sheet, spread the chickpeas out in one layer.

4. Roast the chickpeas for 45 minutes. Check the chickpeas at 30 minutes and monitor closely to prevent burning.

5. Let the chickpeas cool for 10 minutes.

6. Toss the chickpeas in the seasonings and serve.

VARIATION TIP: These roasted chickpeas are easy to customize with a wide variety of flavors. You can spice up this recipe with cayenne pepper. Instead of chili powder and garlic powder, try curry powder and paprika, rosemary and lemon, turmeric and ginger, lemon pepper, cumin and lime, or even cinnamon.

PER SERVING: Calories: 136; Total fat: 4g; Protein: 5g; Carbohydrates: 20g; Fiber: 5g; Sugar: 0g; Sodium: 2mg

SALTY NUT MIX

CONTAINS NUTS AND SEEDS, GLUTEN-FREE, ONE-POT, 30 MINUTES, VEGAN
SERVES 4 / PREP TIME: 5 MINUTES / COOK TIME: 10 MINUTES

This salty nut mix is very low in sodium! The ingredients highlighted in this recipe give the same satisfaction without excess salt. It is recommended to avoid excess sodium on the MIND diet, as well as the Mediterranean and DASH diets. You won't miss the salt in this delicious nut blend.

¼ cup unsalted almonds

¼ cup unsalted shelled pistachios

¼ cup unsalted shelled pumpkin seeds

¼ cup unsalted shelled sunflower seeds

1 teaspoon lemon juice

½ tablespoon lemon pepper

½ tablespoon dried dill weed

¼ teaspoon salt

1. Preheat the oven to 350°F.

2. On a parchment paper–lined baking sheet, spread the nuts in one layer.

3. Roast the nuts for 10 minutes.

4. Let the nuts cool for 10 minutes.

5. Toss the nuts and seeds in the seasonings and serve.

COOKING TIP: This nut mix would go beautifully with a side of tomato slices drizzled in lemon juice and olive oil. Acid and salt enhance each other's flavor, and with just ¼ teaspoon of salt, each serving of this recipe has only 125mg sodium.

PER SERVING: Calories: 209; Total fat: 17g; Protein: 10g; Carbohydrates: 7g; Fiber: 4g; Sugar: 1g; Sodium: 147mg

SPICY NUT MIX

CONTAINS NUTS, GLUTEN-FREE, 30 MINUTES, VEGAN
SERVES 4 / PREP TIME: 5 MINUTES / COOK TIME: 10 MINUTES

This spicy nut mix is crafted with nuts that have a rich, buttery flavor and texture. Cashews, Brazil nuts, macadamia nuts, and pine nuts have a high oil content. The fat in nuts is primarily monounsaturated (healthy) fat, and omega-3 and omega-6 polyunsaturated (healthy) fats. These fats reduce inflammation and improve cardiovascular health, which benefits the brain.

¼ cup unsalted cashews

¼ cup unsalted Brazil nuts

¼ cup unsalted macadamia nuts

¼ cup unsalted pine nuts

½ tablespoon olive oil

½ teaspoon cayenne pepper

1 teaspoon paprika

1 teaspoon dried thyme

1 teaspoon dried oregano

1. Preheat the oven to 350°F.

2. In a large bowl, toss the nuts in the olive oil.

3. On a parchment paper–lined baking sheet, spread the nuts in one layer.

4. Roast the nuts for 10 minutes.

5. Let the nuts cool for 10 minutes.

6. Toss the nuts in the seasonings and serve.

COOKING TIP: Roasting nuts brings out extra richness, flavor, and crunch. The deep-roasted flavor is enhanced by the spices in this blend, and the olive oil helps the spices evenly coat the nuts.

PER SERVING: Calories: 232; Total fat: 23g; Protein: 4g; Carbohydrates: 6g; Fiber: 2g; Sugar: 1g; Sodium: 3mg

SWEET NUT MIX

CONTAINS NUTS, GLUTEN-FREE, ONE-POT, 30 MINUTES, VEGAN
SERVES 4 / PREP TIME: 5 MINUTES / COOK TIME: 10 MINUTES

The dark chocolate and cranberries in this recipe are packed with antioxidants and lend the perfect amount of sweetness to the nuts with no added sugar. Cranberries are rich in vitamin C, manganese, vitamin E, vitamin K, and copper. When dried, cranberries show their sweetness, and when eaten raw they are sour and crisp.

¼ cup unsalted pecans

¼ cup unsalted walnuts

¼ cup unsalted peanuts

¼ cup unsalted hazelnuts

¼ cup vegan dark chocolate chips or chunks

½ cup dried cranberries

1. Preheat the oven to 350°F.

2. On a parchment paper–lined baking sheet, spread the nuts in one layer.

3. Roast the nuts for 8 minutes.

4. Let the nuts cool for 10 minutes.

5. Toss the nuts with the dark chocolate and dried cranberries and serve.

VARIATION TIP: Raisins would also work very well in this nut mix and are sweeter than dried cranberries. If you do not have any dark chocolate, you can toss the nut mix in 1 tablespoon unsweetened cocoa powder for a chocolatey flavor.

PER SERVING: Calories: 313; Total fat: 23g; Protein: 5g; Carbohydrates: 26g; Fiber: 4g; Sugar: 18g; Sodium: 6mg

WHOLE-GRAIN SNACK MIX

CONTAINS NUTS, ONE-POT, 30 MINUTES
SERVES 4 / PREP TIME: 5 MINUTES / COOK TIME: 5 MINUTES

Cereal can be a healthy, whole-grain snack or breakfast. Cereals like Chex, Cheerios, Kellogg's Corn Flakes, and Rice Krispies have little to no added sugar or salt and make a perfect snack. Whole grains are packed with fiber, antioxidants, vitamins, minerals, and even some protein. This mix is a perfect MIND diet snack.

1 cup whole-wheat square cereal (like Chex)

1 cup corn square cereal (like Chex)

1 cup rice square cereal (like Chex)

1 cup toasted O's cereal (like Cheerios)

1 cup peanuts

¼ cup Worcestershire sauce

2 tablespoons olive oil

1 teaspoon paprika

1 teaspoon garlic powder

1 teaspoon onion powder

½ teaspoon cayenne pepper

1. In a large, microwave-safe bowl, toss all the ingredients together until well incorporated.

2. Microwave on high for 2½ minutes, stir, and microwave for another 2½ minutes.

3. Let cool for 10 minutes and serve.

COOKING TIP: You can make this recipe in the oven by baking the mix on baking sheets at 250°F for 1 hour, stirring every 15 minutes.

SUBSTITUTION TIP: Make this mix gluten free by substituting additional rice squares or corn squares for the whole-wheat squares used in this recipe.

PER SERVING: Calories: 215; Total fat: 8g; Protein:4g; Carbohydrates: 35g; Fiber: 4g; Sugar: 6g; Sodium: 460mg

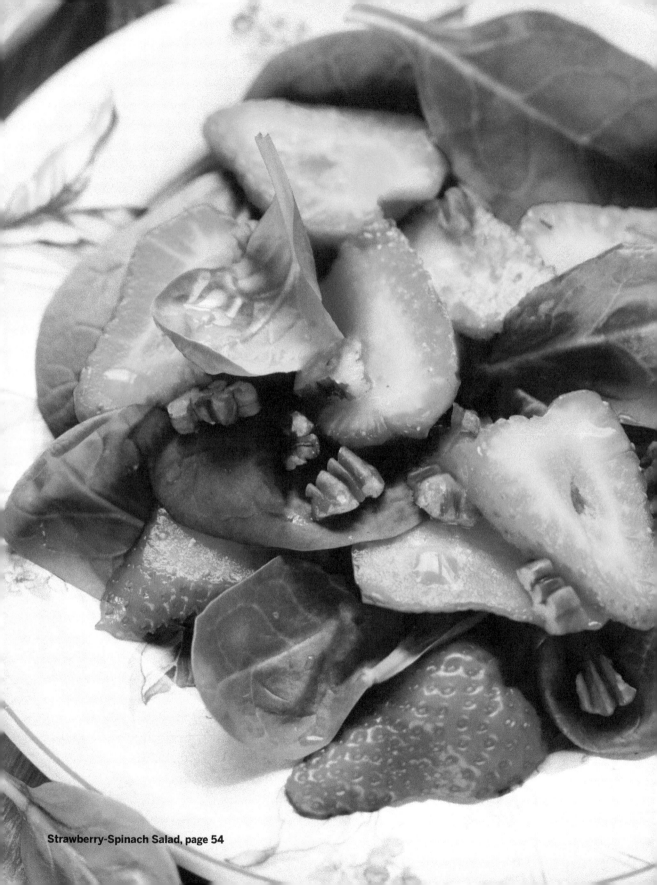

Strawberry-Spinach Salad, page 54

CHAPTER FOUR

SALADS

There are many different types of salads, from simple leafy greens to main dishes with mayonnaise-loaded chicken or tuna to refreshing bowls of mixed fruit. But for the purposes of the MIND diet, a salad is a plant-focused entrée with a variety of proteins, healthy fats, whole grains, and antioxidant-rich fruits. The MIND diet requires one leafy green salad per day, but this does not mean you are married to eating plain lettuce every day for the rest of your life. Salads can be delicious, satisfying, and filled with a wide variety of flavors, textures, and nutrients.

Whole grains such as quinoa or bulgur add additional fiber, vitamins, minerals, and protein to a salad. Nuts add protein, healthy fats, and antioxidants, as well as a crunchy texture. Fruits add important antioxidants, vitamins, and minerals, as well as sweetness and tartness. The dressings in this chapter are made using healthy fats like olive oil, avocado, and nut butter, and they are used sparingly so they don't overpower the salads with excess calories.

RESTAURANT SALADS

Salads are touted as low-calorie, nutrient-rich options for a healthy diet. But while the USDA Food Surveys Research Group reported in 2014 that 20 percent of Americans eat a salad every day, many of those salads have more calories than popular fast foods like a double cheeseburger or pizza. This may seem unbelievable, but burgers at the most popular fast-food restaurants have between 563 and 950 calories, and salads at these same eateries range in calories from 600 to 800 when you include the dressing. Even worse, some salads at certain fast-food restaurants contain more than 1,000 calories! Consumers assume they are making a healthy choice by ordering a salad, but these salads often include fried chicken tenders, high-calorie dressings, cheese, fried chips, and/or fried onions, which not only increase the calorie count but are also loaded with excess sodium, sugar, and cholesterol.

This chapter features great-tasting MIND diet–approved salad recipes that cut down on high-calorie dressings and ingredients. Salads include the Autumn Harvest Salad (page 44), Cranberry-Walnut Broccoli Slaw (page 47), and Vegetable-Quinoa Salad (page 56). Other salads like the Asian-Inspired Chicken Salad (page 43), Cranberry-Chicken Salad (page 46), and Chopped Kale Salad (page 49) add a poultry protein punch. And you can also meet your weekly seafood requirement with the Salmon-Millet Salad (page 51), Salmon Salad Niçoise (page 52), and Warm Salmon and Brussels Sprout Salad (page 57).

ASIAN-INSPIRED CHICKEN SALAD

CONTAINS NUTS, 30 MINUTES

SERVES 2 TO 4 / PREP TIME: 15 MINUTES / COOK TIME: 10 MINUTES

This salad is packed with different flavors and textures and will soon become a staple in your menu rotation. Sweet flavors resonate from the carrots, mandarin oranges, peanut butter, and white wine vinegar. Spice pops from the scallions, bell pepper, ginger, garlic, and red pepper flakes. And just a hint of saltiness is gained from the soy sauce, making a wonderful marriage of flavors commonly found in Asian cuisine.

FOR THE SALAD

1 head napa cabbage

2 scallions, green parts only

1 red bell pepper

2 carrots

1 (15-ounce) can mandarin oranges, drained and rinsed

FOR THE DRESSING

3 tablespoons white wine vinegar

1 teaspoon low-sodium soy sauce

⅓ cup crunchy peanut butter

¼ teaspoon ground ginger

FOR THE CHICKEN

1 teaspoon olive oil

1 pound boneless, skinless chicken breasts, cubed

1 teaspoon minced garlic

1 teaspoon ground ginger

½ teaspoon red pepper flakes

1. Wash and chop the napa cabbage. Set aside.

2. Dice the scallions and bell pepper and shred the carrots. Set aside.

3. In a small bowl, whisk together the vinegar, soy sauce, peanut butter, and ginger. Set aside.

4. In a large sauté pan or skillet, on medium-high heat, heat the olive oil until shimmering.

5. Add the chicken, garlic, ginger, and red pepper flakes. Sauté for 5 to 7 minutes, stirring frequently.

6. On a bed of cabbage, build a salad with the chicken, mandarin oranges, and vegetables. Drizzle the dressing on top and serve.

SUBSTITUTION TIP: Easily make this salad vegan by replacing the chicken with steamed edamame or Crispy Baked Tofu (page 76). Make the dressing gluten-free by replacing the soy sauce with tamari.

PER SERVING: Calories: 685; Total fat: 30g; Protein: 64g; Carbohydrates: 45g; Fiber: 8g; Sugar: 20g; Sodium: 714mg

AUTUMN HARVEST SALAD

GLUTEN-FREE

SERVES 2 TO 4 / PREP TIME: 15 MINUTES / COOK TIME: 30 MINUTES

Fall is one of the best times of the year for produce. The crisp nights give the vegetables a sweetness that is welcomed in this salad. They are high in colorful carotenoids that are powerful antioxidants. This recipe features butternut squash and carrots, which are high in vitamin A, and cabbage and turnips, which are high in vitamin K.

FOR THE SALAD

½ butternut squash, peeled, seeded, and cubed

1 head cauliflower, florets removed

2 turnips, peeled and cubed

2 carrots, sliced

2 tablespoons olive oil

1 teaspoon dried rosemary

1 head cabbage, shredded

FOR THE DRESSING

¼ cup olive oil

2 tablespoons white wine vinegar

1 tablespoon lemon juice

1 teaspoon honey

¼ teaspoon freshly ground black pepper

1. Preheat the oven to 425°F.

2. On a large baking sheet lined with parchment paper, spread the cubed squash, cauliflower florets, turnips, and carrots in a single layer.

3. Drizzle the vegetables with the olive oil and sprinkle with the rosemary.

4. Roast the vegetables for 30 minutes, or until fork-tender.

5. For the dressing, in a small bowl, whisk together the olive oil, vinegar, lemon juice, honey, and pepper.

6. Serve the roasted vegetables on a bed of shredded cabbage, with a drizzle of the dressing.

VARIATION TIP: Any fall vegetables will work well in this salad; check your local produce section for what is on sale—that is what is in season!

PER SERVING: Calories: 680; Total fat: 43g; Protein: 15g; Carbohydrates: 73g; Fiber: 26g; Sugar: 34g; Sodium: 301mg

BLACK BEAN AND CORN SALAD

GLUTEN-FREE, 30 MINUTES

SERVES 2 TO 4 / PREP TIME: 10 MINUTES

Southwest cuisine stems from Native American and Mexican flavors. Core ingredients include beans, corn, and chiles. This salad is a perfect addition to the MIND diet, including recommended servings of both beans and vegetables.

FOR THE DRESSING

1 small avocado, pitted and peeled

2 tablespoons lime juice

⅛ teaspoon cayenne pepper

1 tablespoon honey

FOR THE SALAD

2 (15-ounce) cans no-salt-added black beans, drained and rinsed

1 (15-ounce) can no-salt-added corn, drained

1 red onion, diced

1 red bell pepper, diced

8 cups romaine lettuce, shredded

1. In a blender, purée the avocado, lime juice, cayenne pepper, and honey on high for 30 seconds. Set aside.

2. In a medium bowl, mix the black beans, corn, onion, and red bell pepper.

3. Toss the vegetable mixture in the dressing.

4. Serve the vegetables on a bed of romaine lettuce.

INGREDIENT TIP: The corn chips from chapter 3 (see page 30) would make a great addition to this salad.

SUBSTITUTION TIP: Fresh or frozen corn will work just as well as canned corn.

PER SERVING: Calories: 707; Total fat: 12g; Protein: 35g; Carbohydrates: 123g; Fiber: 32g; Sugar: 28g; Sodium: 47mg

CRANBERRY-CHICKEN SALAD

CONTAINS NUTS, GLUTEN-FREE, 30 MINUTES
SERVES 2 TO 4 / PREP TIME: 15 MINUTES / COOK TIME: 10 MINUTES

This salad is a flavor explosion. Borrowing from Indian cuisine, the chicken is seasoned with cardamom and cinnamon, which pair perfectly with the cranberries. The vinaigrette features cardamom and Dijon mustard, mirroring and enhancing the flavors of the chicken.

FOR THE DRESSING

2 tablespoons olive oil

1 tablespoon white wine vinegar

1 tablespoon Dijon mustard

1 teaspoon ground cardamom

FOR THE CHICKEN

1 teaspoon olive oil

1 pound boneless, skinless chicken breasts, cubed

1 teaspoon ground cardamom

1 teaspoon ground cinnamon

FOR THE SALAD

1 head red leaf romaine lettuce, chopped

1 cup unsweetened dried cranberries

½ cup sliced almonds

1. In a small bowl, whisk together the olive oil, vinegar, mustard, and cardamom. Set aside.

2. In a large sauté pan or skillet, on medium-high heat, heat the olive oil until shimmering.

3. In a large bowl, toss the cubed chicken in the ground cardamom and cinnamon.

4. Add the chicken to the pan and sauté for 5 to 7 minutes, stirring frequently.

5. In a large bowl, toss the lettuce, cranberries, and cooked chicken in the dressing.

6. Serve the salad topped with sliced almonds.

SUBSTITUTION TIP: Fresh cranberries would add a crisp, juicy twist to this salad.

PER SERVING: Calories: 743; Total fat: 34g; Protein: 55g; Carbohydrates: 61g; Fiber: 9g; Sugar: 42g; Sodium: 559mg

CRANBERRY-WALNUT BROCCOLI SLAW

CONTAINS NUTS, GLUTEN-FREE, ONE-POT, 30 MINUTES, VEGAN
SERVES 2 TO 4 / PREP TIME: 10 MINUTES

This salad takes a MIND diet approach to the classic mayonnaise or sour cream–based broccoli slaw. The walnuts provide healthy fat, protein, and omega-3 fatty acids. Broccoli is high in vitamin C and vitamin K as well as folate and potassium. Carrots are a good source of potassium and vitamin K as well as beta carotene, an important antioxidant. Finally, cranberries are rich in vitamin C, vitamin E, vitamin K, and manganese. This salad is a delicious bowl full of antioxidants.

2 large broccoli crowns

2 carrots

1 apple

1 cup unsweetened dried cranberries

½ cup chopped walnuts

¼ cup red wine vinegar

¼ cup olive oil

2 teaspoons onion powder

¼ teaspoon freshly ground black pepper

1. Cut the florets off the stems of broccoli, chop, and put in a large bowl.

2. Over the bowl, grate the broccoli stems and the carrots.

3. Dice the apple and add to the bowl.

4. Add the cranberries, walnuts, vinegar, olive oil, onion powder, and pepper to the bowl and toss. Serve.

INGREDIENT TIP: You can purchase bags of broccoli slaw in the produce section of your local grocer for quicker preparation on a busy night.

PER SERVING: Calories: 720; Total fat: 47g; Protein: 7g; Carbohydrates: 73g; Fiber: 8g; Sugar: 50g; Sodium: 144mg

GREEK SALAD

GLUTEN-FREE, ONE-POT, 30 MINUTES, VEGAN

SERVES 2 TO 4 / PREP TIME: 10 MINUTES

Traditional Greek salad does not include lettuce, but this variation includes mixed spring greens, which make a wonderful addition to a Mediterranean classic. Most likely, any Greek salad you have had has been Americanized. Traditional Greek salad includes only tomato, cucumber, onion, feta, olives, salt, Greek oregano, and olive oil.

1 cucumber, diced

2 Roma tomatoes, diced

1 red onion, diced

1 green bell pepper, diced

1 (15-ounce) can chickpeas, drained and rinsed

¼ cup extra-virgin olive oil

1 tablespoon dried oregano

4 cups mixed spring greens

1. In a large bowl, toss the cucumber, tomatoes, onion, bell pepper, and chickpeas in the olive oil and oregano.

2. Serve on a bed of mixed spring greens.

INGREDIENT TIP: For a bit of extra flavor you can add a few kalamata or green olives. Be careful, though, because they are very high in sodium; 2 olives have over 300mg sodium.

PER SERVING: Calories: 567; Total fat: 30g; Protein: 15g; Carbohydrates: 60g; Fiber: 18g; Sugar: 13g; Sodium: 46mg

CHOPPED KALE SALAD

CONTAINS NUTS, GLUTEN-FREE, 30 MINUTES

SERVES 2 TO 4 / PREP TIME: 10 MINUTES / COOK TIME: 20 MINUTES

Kale is a hearty leafy green rich in B vitamins, antioxidant-rich carotenoids, potassium, calcium, iron, vitamin A, and vitamin C. This salad is a medley of textures from crisp cucumber, creamy avocado, and crunchy pecans. Simple seasonings of basil, pepper, and lemon juice are all this salad needs to reach peak flavor.

32 ounces low-sodium chicken stock

1 tablespoon dried basil, divided

1 teaspoon freshly ground black pepper, divided

1 pound boneless, skinless chicken breasts

¼ cup olive oil

2 tablespoons lemon juice

1 large bunch kale, chopped

1 large tomato, diced

1 cucumber, diced

1 avocado, pitted, peeled, and diced

½ cup pecans

1. In a large sauté pan or skillet, combine the chicken stock, 1½ teaspoons of basil, and ½ teaspoon of black pepper. Bring to a gentle simmer over medium-high heat.

2. Add the chicken and cook for 20 minutes, or until no longer pink in the center and the internal temperature reaches 165°F.

3. In a small bowl, whisk together the olive oil, lemon juice, remaining 1½ teaspoons of basil, and remaining ½ teaspoon of black pepper. Set aside.

4. When the chicken is cooked through, remove from the cooking liquid and shred with 2 forks on a cutting board.

5. On a bed of kale, build a salad with the shredded chicken, tomato, cucumber, avocado, and pecans. Drizzle the dressing on top and serve.

INGREDIENT TIP: A bunch of kale has a lot of sediment in it. Rinse and spin the chopped kale thoroughly to remove all sediment.

SUBSTITUTION TIP: Easily make this salad vegan by replacing the chicken with canned beans of your choice.

PER SERVING: Calories: 979; Total fat: 67g; Protein: 64g; Carbohydrates: 47g; Fiber: 20g; Sugar: 11g; Sodium: 612mg

KALE-SUCCOTASH SALAD

GLUTEN-FREE, VEGAN
SERVES 2 TO 4 / PREP TIME: 10 MINUTES / COOK TIME: 30 MINUTES

Succotash is a corn and shell-bean dish popular in the summer for its refreshing flavors. It is often served with a whole grain and any variety of vegetables on hand. Succotash can be served warm or chilled, and this recipe features it as a hearty salad topping.

1 cup water

1 (15-ounce) can lima beans, drained

1 large bunch kale, chopped

2 ears of corn, kernels removed

1 zucchini, diced

1 cup cherry tomatoes, halved

½ small red onion, diced

2 tablespoons chopped fresh basil

2 tablespoons red wine vinegar

2 tablespoons olive oil

1. In a small pot, bring 1 cup of water to a boil and cook the lima beans for 20 minutes. Drain and set aside to cool for 10 minutes.

2. In a large bowl, mix the lima beans, kale, corn, zucchini, tomatoes, onion, basil, vinegar, and olive oil with tongs. Serve.

INGREDIENT TIP: A bunch of kale has a lot of sediment in it. Rinse and spin the chopped kale thoroughly to remove all sediment.

SUBSTITUTION TIP: If fresh corn is not in season, frozen corn or no-salt-added canned corn also works well.

PER SERVING: Calories: 520; Total fat: 17g; Protein: 23g; Carbohydrates: 48g; Fiber: 27g; Sugar: 17g; Sodium: 698mg

SALMON-MILLET SALAD

GLUTEN-FREE, 30 MINUTES
SERVES 2 TO 4 / PREP TIME: 5 MINUTES / COOK TIME: 20 MINUTES

Millet is a gluten-free whole grain that has a flavor like corn. It is high in calcium, B vitamins, and iron, and is a good source of antioxidants and fiber. Millet is a grain that is not often found in American cooking, but it is a staple in the diets of about one-third of the world's population.

½ cup millet

1 cup water

2 tablespoons olive oil, divided

2 (4-ounce) salmon
fillets, skinless

2 tablespoons Dijon mustard

**2 tablespoons white
wine vinegar**

1 teaspoon honey

4 cups chard or turnip greens

1 cup sugar snap peas

1 broccoli crown, chopped

1. In a microwave-safe bowl, combine the millet and water, and cover the bowl.

2. Microwave on high for 6 to 8 minutes, until all the water is absorbed.

3. In a medium sauté pan or skillet, heat 1 tablespoon of olive oil on medium heat until shimmering.

4. Sear the salmon and cook for 5 minutes, flip, and sear the other side and cook for an additional 5 minutes, until the fish is opaque and flakes easily with a fork.

5. While the salmon is cooking, in a small bowl, whisk together the mustard, vinegar, remaining 1 tablespoon of olive oil, and honey to create the dressing.

6. Serve the turnip greens topped with the salmon, peas, broccoli, and millet, and a drizzle of the dressing.

COOKING TIP: Millet can also be cooked on the stove; the method is the same as for rice: 1 part millet to 2 parts water.

PER SERVING: Calories: 546; Total fat: 21g; Protein: 36g;
Carbohydrates: 54g; Fiber: 13g; Sugar: 10g; Sodium: 1,212mg

SALMON SALAD NIÇOISE

GLUTEN-FREE, 30 MINUTES

SERVES 4 / PREP TIME: 10 MINUTES / COOK TIME: 10 MINUTES

Salad niçoise is a traditional dish from Nice, France. Many variations of preparation exist and are widely disputed by purists. A traditional salad niçoise includes hardboiled egg, tomato, olives, fish, and olive oil. There is great debate about whether the vegetables in a salad niçoise should be raw or cooked.

¼ cup plus 1 tablespoon olive oil

4 (4-ounce) salmon fillets, skinless

8 ounces green beans or string beans

4 small radishes, finely sliced

1 cup grape tomatoes, halved

1 tablespoon whole-grain mustard

4 cups butter lettuce

1 lemon, halved

1. In a medium sauté pan or skillet, heat 1 tablespoon of olive oil on medium heat until shimmering.

2. Pat the salmon fillets dry with paper towels.

3. Sear the salmon and cook on one side for 5 minutes. Flip and sear the other side and cook for 5 additional minutes. The fish should be opaque and flake easily with a fork.

4. In a large bowl, combine the green beans, radishes, and tomatoes with the remaining ¼ cup of olive oil and the mustard and toss together for 10 seconds.

5. Serve the vegetables and the salmon fillets on a bed of butter lettuce, with fresh-squeezed lemon juice on top.

VARIATION TIP: Many Americanized salads niçoise include new potatoes or red potatoes.

PER SERVING: Calories: 325; Total fat: 22g; Protein: 25g; Carbohydrates: 11g; Fiber: 4g; Sugar: 3g; Sodium: 256mg

SOUTHWEST SALAD

GLUTEN-FREE, ONE-POT, 30 MINUTES, VEGAN
SERVES 2 TO 4 / PREP TIME: 10 MINUTES

Southwest cuisine stems from Native American and Mexican flavors, with an American twist. Core ingredients include beans, corn, and chiles. Southwest dishes are plant based, making them perfect additions to the MIND diet, including recommended servings of both beans and vegetables.

¼ cup olive oil

2 tablespoons lime juice

1 tablespoon Mexican dried oregano

1 teaspoon minced garlic

1 (15-ounce) can no-salt-added black beans, drained and rinsed

1 (15-ounce) can no-salt-added pinto beans, drained and rinsed

1 (15-ounce) can no-salt-added corn, drained

1 large tomato, diced

1 jalapeño, diced

1 avocado, pitted, peeled, and diced

1 head iceberg lettuce, shredded

1. In a large bowl, whisk together the olive oil, lime juice, oregano, and garlic to create the dressing.

2. Add the black beans, pinto beans, corn, tomato, jalapeño, and avocado and toss.

3. Serve on a bed of shredded lettuce.

INGREDIENT TIP: The corn chips from chapter 3 (page 30) would make a great addition to this salad.

VARIATION TIP: This salad is vegan but would also work well with leftover chicken or canned tuna.

PER SERVING: Calories: 957; Total fat: 43g; Protein: 34g; Carbohydrates: 118g; Fiber: 33g; Sugar: 21g; Sodium: 63mg

STRAWBERRY-SPINACH SALAD

CONTAINS NUTS, GLUTEN-FREE, ONE-POT, 30 MINUTES, VEGAN
SERVES 2 TO 4 / PREP TIME: 10 MINUTES

Strawberries are antioxidant flavor bombs, just like blueberries, raspberries, and blackberries. They are also great sources of folate, potassium, vitamin C, and manganese. A fun fact is that the most common berries are botanically "false berries" because of the way they grow.

8 cups baby spinach

4 cups strawberries, sliced

½ red onion, thinly sliced

½ cup chopped pecans

¼ cup balsamic vinegar

1. In a large bowl, toss the spinach, strawberries, onion, and pecans together.

2. Drizzle the salad with the balsamic vinegar and serve.

VARIATION TIP: This salad would be delicious with chicken breast, a perfect way to use leftover chicken. Also, sliced almonds would work well in place of the pecans.

PER SERVING: Calories: 359; Total fat: 23g; Protein: 8g; Carbohydrates: 38g; Fiber: 14g; Sugar: 19g; Sodium: 40mg

VEGETABLE-BULGUR SALAD

30 MINUTES, VEGAN

SERVES 2 TO 4 / PREP TIME: 10 MINUTES / COOK TIME: 15 MINUTES

Bulgur, also known as bulgur wheat, is a whole grain popular in Middle Eastern dishes. It makes a nice change from the whole grains more common in American cuisine such as wheat, brown rice, and quinoa. It is particularly high in fiber, folate, and minerals.

FOR THE BULGUR

1 cup water

1 cup bulgur

FOR THE DRESSING

¼ cup olive oil

¼ cup lemon juice

1 teaspoon dried oregano

¼ teaspoon red pepper flakes

FOR THE SALAD

4 cups escarole or mustard greens, packed

1 orange or red bell pepper, diced

1 zucchini, diced

1 cucumber, diced

1 small red onion, diced

1 cup grape tomatoes, halved

1. In a microwave-safe bowl, bring the water to a boil.

2. Add the bulgur to the water and let sit for 7 to 15 minutes, until all the water is absorbed and the grains are tender.

3. For the dressing, in a small bowl, whisk together the olive oil, lemon juice, oregano and red pepper flakes.

4. Serve a salad of greens topped with the bell pepper, zucchini, cucumber, onion, tomatoes, and bulgur, drizzled with the dressing.

COOKING TIP: The bulgur most commonly found in stores will need to be soaked for 7 to 15 minutes. Coarsely ground bulgur is harder to find but can be cooked without soaking.

PER SERVING: Calories: 611; Total fat: 30g; Protein: 19g; Carbohydrates: 80g; Fiber: 24g; Sugar: 14g; Sodium: 79mg

VEGETABLE-QUINOA SALAD

GLUTEN-FREE, 30 MINUTES
SERVES 2 TO 4 / PREP TIME: 10 MINUTES / COOK TIME: 20 MINUTES

Quinoa is a unique plant. It is a complete plant protein, containing all nine essential amino acids. Most other plant proteins need to be paired together to create a complete protein. As a whole grain, quinoa is high in fiber, vitamins, and minerals. As if protein and whole grains were not enough in one food, quinoa also contains antioxidants. It is a true superfood.

2 cups water

1 cup quinoa, rinsed

1 yellow bell pepper

1 large leek, well rinsed

1 head purple cabbage

1 (15-ounce) can no-salt-added chickpeas, drained and rinsed

2 tablespoons olive oil

2 tablespoons lime juice

1 teaspoon ground cumin

1 tablespoon chopped fresh cilantro

1. In a medium pot, bring the water to a boil.

2. Add the quinoa to the boiling water, reduce the heat to low, cover, and simmer for 20 minutes, or until the quinoa can be fluffed with a fork.

3. While the quinoa is cooking, dice the bell pepper, slice the leek, and shred the cabbage.

4. In a large bowl, mix the quinoa, bell pepper, leek, cabbage, chickpeas, olive oil, lime juice, cumin, and cilantro for 30 seconds. Serve.

COOKING TIP: Rinsing the quinoa before cooking will ensure no debris makes its way into your meal.

PER SERVING: Calories: 868; Total fat: 23g; Protein: 31g; Carbohydrates: 142g; Fiber: 30g; Sugar: 26g; Sodium: 106mg

WARM SALMON AND BRUSSELS SPROUT SALAD

CONTAINS NUTS, GLUTEN-FREE, 30 MINUTES

SERVES 4 / PREP TIME: 10 MINUTES / COOK TIME: 10 MINUTES

Brussels sprouts are from the cabbage family and originate in the Mediterranean. While we normally see them as tiny cabbages at the grocery store, they actually grow on large stalks. They are very high in vitamin C, vitamin K, antioxidants, and fiber. They also contain omega-3 fatty acids, which work to reduce inflammation.

2 tablespoons olive oil, divided

4 (4-ounce) salmon fillets, skinless

1 pound Brussels sprouts, shredded or chopped

1 cup fresh cranberries

8 ounces endive, chopped

1 lemon, halved

¼ cup unsalted pecan pieces

1. In a medium sauté pan or skillet, heat 1 tablespoon of olive oil on medium heat until shimmering.

2. At the same time, in a large sauté pan or skillet, heat the remaining 1 tablespoon of olive oil on medium heat until shimmering.

3. Pat the salmon fillets dry with paper towels.

4. In the first (medium) pan, sear the salmon on one side and cook for 5 minutes. Flip and sear the other side and cook for 5 additional minutes. The fish should be opaque and flake easily with a fork.

5. In the second (large) pan, sauté the Brussels sprouts, cranberries, and endive for 10 minutes, stirring frequently.

6. Serve the salmon on top of the vegetables and cranberries, with a squeeze of fresh lemon juice and pecan pieces on top.

VARIATION TIP: This salad can also be made with raw vegetables, with cooked salmon on top.

PER SERVING: Calories: 252; Total fat: 14g; Protein: 15g; Carbohydrates: 19g; Fiber: 9g; Sugar: 4g; Sodium: 80mg

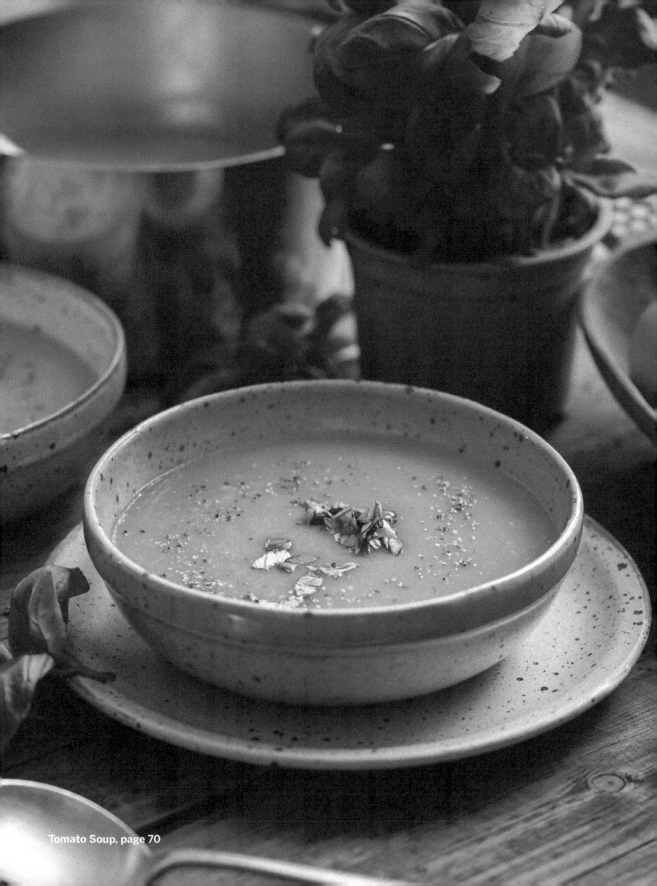

Tomato Soup, page 70

CHAPTER FIVE

SOUPS AND STEWS

F or many of us, soup provides warmth and comfort in one time-saving bowl of goodness. It is such a treat after a full week of cooking to be able to throw leftover ingredients into a slow cooker, forget about it, and sit down to a satisfying bowl of soup. Dipping a crusty piece of bread in flavorful broth or a bowl of stew feels very rewarding. The secret is that the best soups do not come out of a can, but rather out of your kitchen.

The MIND diet recommends incorporating a lot of different vegetables in your daily meals, and the soups and stews in this chapter will make it easy to meet those requirements. Vegetables are excellent sources of the vitamins, minerals, and antioxidants that are at the heart of the MIND diet.

MIND IN A BOWL

Soups and stews can be rich in vitamins, minerals, and nutrients and a great way to satisfy multiple MIND diet food requirements in one bowl. The MIND diet recommends eating three servings of whole grains and one (nonsalad) serving of vegetables per day, eating ½ cup of beans or legumes 3 to 4 times per week, having poultry at least twice per week, and using olive oil for cooking. Each of the great-tasting soup and stew recipes that follow meet two or more of these MIND diet requirements.

Enjoy meeting your poultry and bean requirements with the White Bean and Chicken Chili (page 71), Chicken Tortilla Soup (page 64), and Slow-Cooker White Bean, Chicken, and Kale Soup (page 67). Fulfill your vegetable and legume requirements with Black Bean Soup (page 61), Lentil Rice Soup (page 65), Split Pea Soup (page 68), and Sweet Potato, Collard Greens, and Black-Eyed Pea Soup (page 69). Check off a poultry, whole-grain, and vegetable requirement with Chicken-Quinoa Stew over Sweet Potatoes (page 62). Finally, get extra servings of vegetables and show off olive oil's versatility with Tomato Soup (page 70) and Refrigerator-Cleaner Soup (page 66).

BLACK BEAN SOUP

GLUTEN-FREE, VEGAN

SERVES 4 / PREP TIME: 10 MINUTES / COOK TIME: 40 MINUTES

Black beans are an important food on the MIND diet, along with any other bean or legume of your liking. They are fiber rich and full of antioxidants, as well as protein! Serving for serving, black beans are actually higher in protein than meat, and they have no cholesterol. One cup of black beans has more protein than a chicken leg.

1 small white onion, finely diced

1 red bell pepper, diced

2 tablespoons olive oil

4 (15-ounce) cans no-salt-added black beans, undrained

1 cup low-sodium vegetable stock

1 teaspoon ground cumin

1 teaspoon garlic powder

1 teaspoon dried oregano

1 tablespoon lime juice

1. In a large pot over medium heat, sauté the onion and bell pepper in the olive oil for 10 minutes.

2. Add the black beans and their juices, vegetable stock, cumin, garlic powder, oregano, and lime juice and simmer for 30 minutes.

3. In a blender or food processor, use the pulse button to blend half of the soup in 10-second increments, until a smooth but thick consistency is reached.

4. Add the blended soup back into the remaining mixture, stir together, and serve.

COOKING TIP: If you prefer a chunky soup, you do not have to purée any of the soup. If you prefer a thinner soup, you can purée the entire batch.

SUBSTITUTION TIP: If you prefer to use dried beans over canned, simply soak the beans in water overnight, or all day when you are at work, and they will be ready to go into this recipe.

PER SERVING: Calories: 470; Total fat: 11g; Protein: 25g; Carbohydrates: 71g; Fiber: 26g; Sugar: 2g; Sodium: 1,316mg

CHICKEN-QUINOA STEW OVER SWEET POTATOES

GLUTEN-FREE

SERVES 4 / PREP TIME: 15 MINUTES / COOK TIME: 40 MINUTES

A sweet potato adds a sweetness, earthy flavor, and creamy texture to this stew. Leaving the skin on the sweet potato retains all the vitamins and minerals that are beneficial to your health. Sweet potatoes are extremely high in vitamin A and are a great source of vitamin C, potassium, and vitamin B_6. Best of all, sweet potatoes are rich in antioxidants and reduce inflammation.

1 large sweet potato, washed, with skin on

2 tablespoons olive oil, divided

2 cups water

1 cup quinoa, rinsed

1 pound boneless, skinless chicken breasts, cubed

1 (15-ounce) can no-salt-added black beans, drained and rinsed

20 ounces low-sodium chicken stock

2 teaspoons ground cumin

2 teaspoons chili powder

2 teaspoons garlic powder

2 teaspoons onion powder

½ teaspoon cayenne pepper

1. Preheat the oven to 450°F.

2. While the oven is preheating, cube the sweet potato.

3. On a baking sheet lined with parchment paper, lay the sweet potato cubes in a single layer and drizzle with the olive oil.

4. Roast the sweet potato cubes for 30 minutes, flipping the cubes halfway.

5. While the sweet potatoes are cooking, in a medium pot, bring the water to a boil.

6. Add the quinoa to the boiling water, reduce the heat to low, cover, and simmer for 20 minutes, until the quinoa can be fluffed with a fork.

7. While the quinoa is cooking, in a large pot or deep pan, heat the remaining olive oil and brown the cubed chicken.

8. Add the black beans, chicken stock, cumin, chili powder, garlic powder, onion powder, and cayenne pepper to the browned chicken and bring to a low boil. Allow to simmer for 10 minutes.

9. Just prior to serving, stir the quinoa into the chicken and black bean soup mixture.

10. Ladle the stew over the sweet potato and serve.

COOKING TIP: This stew can also be made in a slow cooker. Simply add all the ingredients to a slow cooker and cook on high for 3 to 4 hours.

PER SERVING: Calories: 471; Total fat: 10g; Protein: 37g; Carbohydrates: 61g; Fiber: 10g; Sugar: 8g; Sodium: 295mg

CHICKEN TORTILLA SOUP

GLUTEN-FREE, ONE-POT, SLOW COOKER
SERVES 4 / PREP TIME: 10 MINUTES / COOK TIME: 4 HOURS

Tortilla soup is a classic of Mexican cuisine that fits in perfectly on the MIND diet. This variation contains no added salt and is rich in legumes and vegetables. This recipe is designed with mild spice and can be spiced up to your liking with hotter chiles or jalapeños or with a dash of hot sauce when serving.

1 pound boneless, skinless chicken breasts

32 ounces low-sodium chicken stock

1 (15-ounce) can no-salt-added black beans, drained and rinsed

1 (15-ounce) can no-salt-added pinto beans, drained and rinsed

1 (15-ounce) can no-salt-added corn, drained

1 (4-ounce) can diced mild green chiles or mild jalapeños, drained

1 (15-ounce) can no-salt-added diced tomatoes, drained

1 (1.25-ounce) packet salt-free taco seasoning, like Mrs. Dash

1 bunch cilantro, stemmed and coarsely chopped

1. In a slow cooker, combine the whole chicken breasts and chicken stock.

2. Cover and cook on high for 2 hours.

3. Strain the fat from the broth with a slotted spoon or mesh strainer.

4. Add the black beans, pinto beans, corn, chiles, tomatoes, and taco seasoning, cover, and cook on high for 2 more hours.

5. Remove the chicken breasts and shred with 2 forks on a cutting board.

6. Return the shredded chicken to the soup.

7. Serve each bowl of soup topped with a sprinkle of cilantro.

COOKING TIP: This chicken tortilla soup would be perfect topped with corn chips, guacamole, or salsa (page 30).

PER SERVING: Calories: 418; Total fat: 5g; Protein: 41g; Carbohydrates: 58g; Fiber: 14g; Sugar: 10g; Sodium: 466mg

LENTIL RICE SOUP

GLUTEN-FREE, ONE-POT, VEGAN
SERVES 4 / PREP TIME: 10 MINUTES / COOK TIME: 1 HOUR

Lentils are legumes that have long been a staple in the diets of many cultures. Brown lentils have the mildest flavor and are the most commonly used. Green lentils have a peppery flavor, red lentils have a nutty flavor, yellow lentils are sweeter, and black lentils have a robust flavor and are heartier. Lentils are rich in fiber, protein, vitamins, and minerals. Pairing lentils with rice results in a complete vegan protein.

2 cups dried brown lentils

1 cup wild rice

5 carrots, coarsely chopped

8 cups water

2 bay leaves

1 teaspoon dried thyme

1 teaspoon garlic powder

2 cups baby spinach

1 lemon, halved

1. In a large stockpot, combine the lentils, wild rice, carrots, water, bay leaves, thyme, and garlic powder.

2. Bring to a boil.

3. Reduce the heat and simmer for 1 hour.

4. During the last few minutes before serving, stir in the spinach and allow to wilt.

5. Remove the bay leaves, top with fresh-squeezed lemon juice, and serve.

COOKING TIP: Rinse lentils in a strainer to remove any sediment and check for any small rocks or debris.

PER SERVING: Calories: 508; Total fat: 2g; Protein: 31g; Carbohydrates: 94g; Fiber: 31g; Sugar: 8g; Sodium: 75mg

REFRIGERATOR-CLEANER SOUP

GLUTEN-FREE, VEGAN
SERVES 4 / PREP TIME: 10 MINUTES / COOK TIME: 35 MINUTES

This soup is the perfect way to use up any leftover vegetables from the week, even if they are starting to get soft or have wilted. With potatoes as the base, this soup has body and creaminess. Any vegetables can be used to lend this soup color and flavor.

3 medium potatoes

1 small onion

2 carrots

2 celery stalks

1 bunch asparagus, trimmed

1 tablespoon olive oil

32 ounces low-sodium vegetable stock

Freshly ground black pepper

2 tablespoons chopped fresh parsley

1 cup unsweetened plain nondairy milk

1. Coarsely chop the potatoes, onion, carrots, celery, and asparagus.

2. In a stockpot or a large and deep sauté pan or skillet, sauté all the vegetables in the olive oil over medium heat for 10 minutes.

3. Add the vegetable stock, pepper, and parsley. Cover and simmer for 25 minutes.

4. Purée in a blender in 4 batches, with ¼ cup of nondairy milk in each batch, and serve.

INGREDIENT TIP: Leave the skins on the potatoes for extra fiber, vitamins, and minerals. Because this soup is puréed, you will never notice the skins.

SUBSTITUTION TIP: This soup would be just as delicious with squash, broccoli, peppers, leafy greens, or any fresh herbs that might be wilting.

PER SERVING: Calories: 212; Total fat: 5g; Protein: 6g; Carbohydrates: 38g; Fiber: 8g; Sugar: 7g; Sodium: 185mg

SLOW-COOKER WHITE BEAN, CHICKEN, AND KALE SOUP

GLUTEN-FREE, ONE-POT, SLOW COOKER

SERVES 4 / PREP TIME: 10 MINUTES / COOK TIME: 3 HOURS

Depending on how much broth you prefer, you can make this recipe into a chili, stew, or soup. Kale is a hearty green that holds up well in soup preparations, retaining a meaty chew rather than falling apart.

1 pound boneless, skinless chicken breasts

32 ounces low-sodium chicken stock

2 (15-ounce) cans no-salt-added great northern beans or cannellini beans, drained and rinsed

2 celery stalks, chopped

2 carrots, chopped

1 tablespoon chopped fresh parsley

½ tablespoon dried oregano

1 teaspoon garlic powder

1 teaspoon onion powder

½ bunch kale, thoroughly rinsed and dried, coarsely chopped

1. In a slow cooker, combine all the ingredients. Cover and cook on high for 3 hours.

2. Remove the chicken from the slow cooker and shred using 2 forks on a cutting board.

3. Return the chicken to the slow cooker, stir into the soup, and serve.

INGREDIENT TIP: For a crunchy twist on this soup, bake Kale Chips (page 32) and serve on top of the soup, rather than boiling the kale in the soup itself.

PER SERVING: Calories: 353; Total fat: 5g; Protein: 37g; Carbohydrates: 43g; Fiber: 15g; Sugar: 3g; Sodium: 519mg

SPLIT PEA SOUP

SERVES 4 / PREP TIME: 10 MINUTES / COOK TIME: 4 TO 5 HOURS

Split peas are from a family called legumes, which are pod vegetables with edible seeds. Other examples of legumes include soybeans, peanuts, lentils, and lima beans. Split pea soup is the dish that most commonly comes to mind when cooking with split peas, but you can also make split pea fritters, crispy split peas, or curry.

2 medium potatoes, scrubbed

1 small onion

3 carrots

1 (16-ounce) package green split peas

32 ounces low-sodium vegetable stock

1 cup water

Freshly ground black pepper

1. Coarsely chop the potatoes, onion, and carrots.

2. In a slow cooker, combine the potatoes, onion, carrots, split peas, vegetable stock, and water.

3. Cover and cook on high for 4 to 5 hours, until the split peas have begun to break down.

4. Season with black pepper and serve.

VARIATION TIP: This is a delicious vegan recipe that can be just as delicious if you add chunks of cooked chicken or turkey. Yellow split peas can also be used in this recipe. They will have an earthier flavor than the sweeter green peas.

PER SERVING: Calories: 406; Total fat: <1g; Protein: 32g; Carbohydrates: 93g; Fiber: 33g; Sugar: 15g; Sodium: 140mg

SWEET POTATO, COLLARD GREENS, AND BLACK-EYED PEA SOUP

GLUTEN-FREE, ONE-POT, VEGAN

SERVES 4 / PREP TIME: 10 MINUTES / COOK TIME: 40 MINUTES

Black-eyed peas are a Southern staple, often served with collard greens. These legumes are a great variety to include on the MIND diet, as part of bean intake at least three times per week.

1 large sweet potato, washed and cubed

1 (15-ounce) can no-salt-added black-eyed peas, drained and rinsed

1 (15-ounce) can no-salt-added crushed tomatoes

½ bunch collard greens, rinsed, stemmed, and chopped

32 ounces low-sodium vegetable stock

1 tablespoon dried oregano

1 teaspoon garlic powder

1 tablespoon smoked paprika

In a large stockpot, cook all the ingredients on high for 40 minutes, until the sweet potatoes are tender.

COOKING TIP: Cubed sweet potatoes can also be roasted in the oven for 30 to 40 minutes until tender and added to the soup before serving, to add a different texture to the soup. Roasted sweet potatoes have a chewy to crisp skin and tender flesh inside. Alternatively, the soup can be served over a baked sweet potato.

PER SERVING: Calories: 182; Total fat: 1g; Protein: 8g; Carbohydrates: 35g; Fiber: 9g; Sugar: 12g; Sodium: 156mg

TOMATO SOUP

GLUTEN-FREE, 30 MINUTES, VEGAN
SERVES 2 TO 4 / PREP TIME: 10 MINUTES / COOK TIME: 20 MINUTES

This simple tomato soup requires very little seasoning, allowing the robust flavor of the cherry tomatoes and red bell peppers to shine through. The garlic and olive oil add just enough richness to cut through the acid from the vegetables, and the soup has a natural sweetness from the cherry tomatoes.

2 red bell peppers

4 cups cherry tomatoes

1 tablespoon minced garlic

2 tablespoons olive oil, plus more for serving

32 ounces low-sodium vegetable stock

½ cup chopped fresh parsley

1. Preheat the oven to 400°F.

2. While the oven is preheating, halve the bell peppers and remove the seeds and ribs.

3. On a parchment paper–lined baking sheet, spread the tomatoes and bell pepper halves in a single layer. Evenly sprinkle with the minced garlic and drizzle with the olive oil.

4. Roast the vegetables for 20 minutes, turning after 10 minutes to prevent burning.

5. Transfer the vegetables to a blender and add the vegetable stock. Blend on high, or purée for 30 to 60 seconds.

6. Drizzle each bowl of soup with olive oil, sprinkle with the fresh parsley, and serve.

COOKING TIP: I almost always recommend lining baking sheets with parchment paper. This simple step makes cleanup a breeze.

SUBSTITUTION TIP: In place of the cherry tomatoes, hot-house tomatoes, beefsteak tomatoes, or Roma tomatoes would work equally well.

PER SERVING: Calories: 256; Total fat: 15g; Protein: 4g; Carbohydrates: 28g; Fiber: 6g; Sugar: 13g; Sodium: 188mg

WHITE BEAN AND CHICKEN CHILI

GLUTEN-FREE, ONE-POT

SERVES 4 / PREP TIME: 10 MINUTES / COOK TIME: 40 MINUTES

This chili has a kick from the diced green chiles. Green chiles are a great source of beta carotene, a carotenoid antioxidant, and an excellent source of vitamin C. Green chiles have a unique flavor profile with sweetness, spiciness, and smokiness.

1 tablespoon olive oil

1 pound boneless, skinless chicken breasts, diced

2 (15-ounce) cans no-salt-added great northern beans or cannellini beans, drained

1 (15-ounce) can no-salt-added diced tomatoes

1 (7-ounce) can diced mild green chiles, drained

2 teaspoons chili powder

2 teaspoons dried oregano

16 ounces low-sodium chicken stock

1 medium avocado, pitted, peeled, and sliced

1 bunch cilantro, stemmed

1. In a large stockpot, heat the olive oil over medium heat and brown the diced chicken.

2. Add the beans, diced tomatoes, green chiles, chili powder, oregano, and chicken stock.

3. Cook on medium-high heat for 30 minutes.

4. Serve with avocado slices and cilantro.

INGREDIENT TIP: Cilantro is the same plant from which we get coriander seeds.

SUBSTITUTION TIP: For a spicier chili, use medium or hot diced green chiles or jalapeños.

PER SERVING: Calories: 466; Total fat: 13g; Protein: 41g; Carbohydrates: 51g; Fiber: 17g; Sugar: 8g; Sodium: 565mg

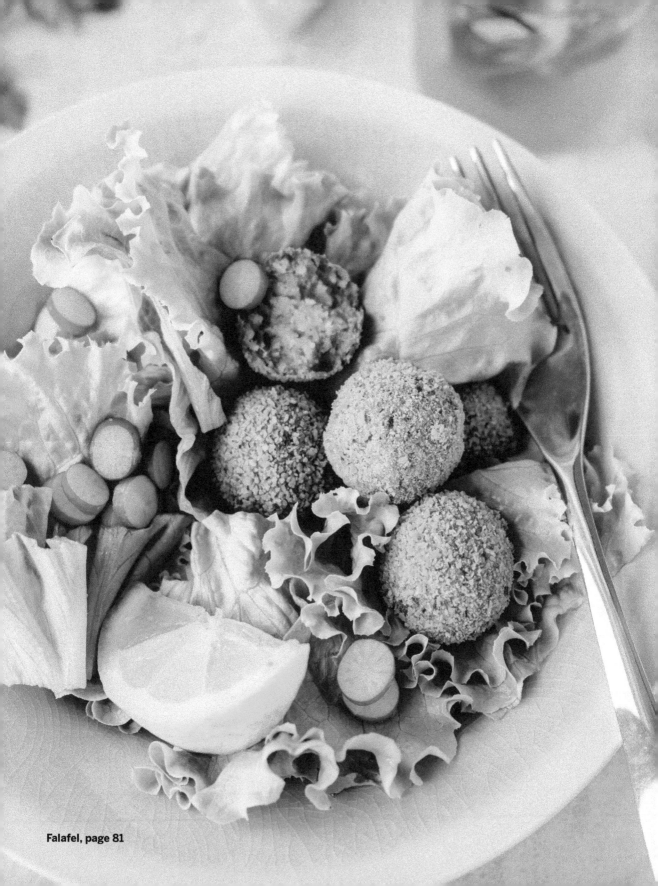

Falafel, page 81

VEGAN ENTRÉES

ncorporating vegan dishes into your diet does not mean you have to become a vegan. Vegan dishes are delicious ways to ensure that you are meeting your vegetable requirements on the MIND diet. Veganism is a diet containing no animal products, meaning no meat, seafood, or animal by-products like eggs, milk, butter, or cheese.

Vegan dishes rely on plant-based proteins like beans and legumes, nuts and nut butters, seeds, tofu and soybeans, and whole grains. For the purposes of the MIND diet, vegan dishes can be served with poultry and seafood, which provide their own important health benefits for delaying or preventing cognitive decline.

SODIUM AND SUGAR IN VEGETABLES

According to USDA researchers, the average American eats 1½ cups of vegetables a day, about half of what the *Dietary Guidelines for Americans* recommends. Furthermore, the same researchers found that half of the average American's vegetable intake comes from potatoes and tomatoes—both of which, though healthy in their natural states, are usually prepared with lots of unhealthy additives like sugar, salt, cream, butter, and cheese!

The recipes in this chapter celebrate vegetables as they are, using fresh complementary flavors instead of excess sugar and salt for seasoning. Examples of the minimal amounts of added sugar in these recipes include 1 tablespoon of agave syrup in the Crispy Baked Tofu (page 76), 3 grams of added sugar per 1 tablespoon of low-sodium soy sauce in the Tofu Stir-Fry (page 90), and 4 grams of added sugar per ¼ cup of peanut butter in the Asian-Inspired Peanut Noodles (page 75).

ASIAN-INSPIRED PEANUT NOODLES

CONTAINS NUTS, 30 MINUTES, VEGAN
SERVES 4 / PREP TIME: 10 MINUTES / COOK TIME: 15 MINUTES

Peanuts are widely used in Asian cooking. Peanut sauces vary from sweet to spicy, thick to thin, and are served as dipping sauces and on pasta, meats, and vegetables. Peanuts are high in protein, omega-6 fatty acids, and a plethora of vitamins and minerals, making them a great food for the MIND diet.

4 cups water

8 ounces whole-wheat spaghetti

2 tablespoons olive oil

1 red bell pepper, sliced

¼ cup crunchy peanut butter

3 tablespoons low-sodium soy sauce

2 tablespoons white wine vinegar

½ tablespoon ground ginger

2 scallions, green parts only, sliced

1. In a large pot, bring the water to a boil.

2. Boil the pasta for 10 to 12 minutes, until tender. Drain.

3. In a medium sauté pan or skillet, heat the olive oil on low heat. Add the bell pepper, peanut butter, soy sauce, vinegar, and ginger and cook, stirring, for 10 minutes.

4. Add the pasta to the sauce and mix thoroughly.

5. Serve with the scallions sprinkled on top.

VARIATION TIP: Add tofu to this recipe for an extra boost of protein. Also make this recipe gluten-free by substituting rice noodles and tamari for the spaghetti and soy sauce.

PER SERVING: Calories: 359; Total fat: 18g; Protein: 11g; Carbohydrates: 48g; Fiber: 8g; Sugar: 2g; Sodium: 495mg

CRISPY BAKED TOFU

VEGAN

SERVES 2 TO 4 / PREP TIME: 1 HOUR / COOK TIME: 40 MINUTES

Tofu is a versatile vegan protein that can take on a variety of textures and flavors. From silken tofu in smoothies to this crispy baked tofu, there is a place for this bean curd in every diet, barring a soy allergy.

14 ounces extra-firm tofu

1 tablespoon low-sodium soy sauce

1 tablespoon agave syrup

1 tablespoon lemon juice

1 tablespoon minced garlic

½ teaspoon ground ginger

1. Line a plate with several paper towels. Remove the tofu block from the package and place on the paper towels.

2. Add additional paper towels on top of the tofu block and place a cutting board on top of the paper towels.

3. Weigh the cutting board down with a heavy book, a pot, or several cans.

4. Leave the tofu to drain for at least 30 minutes.

5. Cut the tofu into 1-inch cubes.

6. Preheat the oven to 350°F.

7. In a large bowl, whisk together the marinade of soy sauce, agave syrup, lemon juice, garlic, and ginger.

8. Marinate the tofu for 30 minutes.

9. On a parchment paper–lined baking sheet, place the tofu in a single layer.

10. Bake for 20 minutes, flip the cubes, and bake for 20 minutes more. Serve.

COOKING TIP: You can also fry the tofu in a pan with hot oil. Baking the tofu takes a bit longer but requires no oil and requires less monitoring.

SUBSTITUTION TIP: Substitute tamari for the soy sauce to make this dish gluten-free.

PER SERVING: Calories: 233; Total fat: 9g; Protein: 22g; Carbohydrates: 18g; Fiber: 3g; Sugar: 9g; Sodium: 349mg

EGGPLANT-TOFU LASAGNA

GLUTEN-FREE, VEGAN
SERVES 2 TO 4 / PREP TIME: 30 MINUTES / COOK TIME: 40 MINUTES

Eggplant is a nightshade fruit that is often used in vegan cooking as a meat substitute. In this preparation it takes the place of the pasta. Eggplants are high in antioxidants, particularly the anthocyanin that gives them their deep color. Fun fact: Eggplant is technically a fruit, just like tomatoes, and is closely related to blueberries!

14 ounces regular or firm tofu

2 medium eggplants

1 (15-ounce) can no-salt-added tomato sauce

1 tablespoon Italian seasoning

2 teaspoons garlic powder

2 teaspoons onion powder

¼ teaspoon chili powder

1. Line a plate with several paper towels. Remove the tofu block from the package and place on the paper towels.

2. Add additional paper towels on top of the tofu block and place a cutting board on top of the paper towels.

3. Weigh the cutting board down with a heavy book, a pot, or several cans.

4. Leave the tofu to drain for at least 30 minutes.

5. Preheat the oven to 375°F.

6. While the tofu is being pressed, peel and cut the eggplants into ¼-inch-thick slices horizontally or vertically.

7. Allow the eggplant slices to drain on several layers of paper towels for 15 minutes to remove excess moisture.

8. On a parchment paper–lined baking sheet, place the eggplant slices in a single layer. Bake for 10 minutes, flip, and bake for 10 more minutes.

9. While the eggplant is baking, in a small bowl, mix the tomato sauce, Italian seasoning, garlic powder, onion powder, and chili powder; set aside.

10. In a medium bowl, crumble the tofu into small kernels using your fingers; set aside.

11. In a large baking dish, layer a spoonful of tomato sauce, then a layer of eggplant, then a layer of tofu crumbles. Repeat until all the eggplant and tofu have been used.

12. Top with one final layer of tomato sauce.

13. Bake for 30 minutes.

14. Remove the lasagna from the oven and allow to rest for 10 minutes. Cut and serve while hot.

VARIATION TIP: Zucchini slices can be used in place of the eggplant; simply skip steps 7 and 8.

PER SERVING: Calories: 405; Total fat: 11g; Protein: 28g; Carbohydrates: 56g; Fiber: 21g; Sugar: 27g; Sodium: 147mg

CAULIFLOWER STEAKS

GLUTEN-FREE, ONE-POT, 30 MINUTES, VEGAN
SERVES 2 TO 4 / PREP TIME: 5 MINUTES / COOK TIME: 10 MINUTES

Cauliflower is a wonderfully versatile vegetable that is used frequently in vegan cooking. You can "rice" the cauliflower by grating it and use it as a rice or ground meat substitute, and, due to its firmness, it gives a meaty texture to many dishes. It is high in antioxidants, B vitamins, choline, and fiber. These cauliflower "steaks" can be served on a bun like a burger, over a bed of quinoa or brown rice, or with a ladle full of stew on top.

2 tablespoons olive oil

2 cauliflower crowns

Freshly ground black pepper

1. In a large sauté pan or skillet, heat the olive oil on medium heat until shimmering.

2. Slice down the crown of each cauliflower through the stem, to yield two halves of the cauliflower. Slice off the tapered ends of the cauliflower, leaving 4 large steaks.

3. Season the cauliflower steaks with black pepper.

4. Sear the cauliflower for 3 to 5 minutes per side, until golden brown.

5. Serve as the base of any dish of your choice.

VARIATION TIP: This is a basic recipe with minimal seasoning. Flavor your cauliflower steaks to match your meal by adding spices like garlic, red pepper flakes, or Italian seasoning.

PER SERVING: Calories: 153; Total fat: 14g; Protein: 3g; Carbohydrates: 7g; Fiber: 3g; Sugar: 3g; Sodium: 40mg

FALAFEL

30 MINUTES, VEGAN

SERVES 2 TO 4 / PREP TIME: 10 MINUTES / COOK TIME: 10 MINUTES

Falafel is a Middle Eastern staple made from ground legumes, onion, herbs, and spices. These fried fritters are a very popular vegan favorite because of their savory flavor and the crispy exterior wrapped around a soft middle. The combination of ingredients checks off several requirements on the MIND diet. Serve the falafel atop salad or on pita bread.

2 (15-ounce) cans chickpeas, drained and rinsed

½ onion, coarsely chopped

1 cup fresh parsley leaves

¼ cup minced garlic

¼ cup all-purpose flour

1 teaspoon ground cumin

1 tablespoon lemon juice

¼ cup olive oil

1. In a blender or food processor, combine the chickpeas with the onion, parsley, garlic, flour, cumin, and lemon juice. Pulse until the mixture has a fine texture, but with some chunks remaining, 30 seconds to 1 minute.

2. In a large sauté pan or skillet, heat the olive oil on medium heat until shimmering.

3. Make each falafel by shaping 2 tablespoons of the mixture into a ball, then flattening into a disk, about 2 inches in diameter.

4. Fry the falafel in the pan for 4 minutes, flipping and cooking for 4 minutes more, or until golden brown. Serve.

SUBSTITUTION TIP: Make this recipe gluten-free by using your favorite gluten-free flour.

VARIATION TIP: Fava beans are also commonly used in falafel and can be used in place of the chickpeas.

COOKING TIP: You can also make this recipe in the oven by baking the falafel at 350°F for 20 minutes, flipping them halfway through cooking.

PER SERVING: Calories: 761; Total fat: 31g; Protein: 25g; Carbohydrates: 99g; Fiber: 24g; Sugar: 2g; Sodium: 24mg

LENTIL CURRY

GLUTEN-FREE, VEGAN
SERVES 2 TO 4 / PREP TIME: 10 MINUTES / COOK TIME: 40 MINUTES

Curry is a traditional Indian cooking preparation of stewing spices in a sauce. Types of curries vary by geographical location, culture, and food preferences. Curries can be soups, stews, vegetarian, vegan, or include meat or seafood. The influence of curry has spread worldwide, and every culture has its own variation. Serve alone, over rice, or with naan.

1 cup red lentils

2 cups water

2 tablespoons olive oil

½ yellow onion, minced

3 tablespoons minced garlic '

1 (15-ounce) can no-salt-added crushed tomatoes

1½ cups low-sodium vegetable stock

2 tablespoons curry powder or curry paste

1 teaspoon ground ginger

1 teaspoon ground turmeric

1 teaspoon ground cumin

¼ teaspoon ground allspice

1. In a medium pot, bring the lentils and water to a boil.

2. Reduce the heat to medium-low and cover the pot. Simmer for 20 minutes.

3. In a large and deep sauté pan or skillet, heat the olive oil on medium heat until shimmering.

4. Sauté the onion and garlic for 10 minutes.

5. Add the crushed tomatoes, vegetable stock, curry powder, ginger, turmeric, cumin, and allspice to the onion-and-garlic mixture and simmer for 10 more minutes.

6. Drain the lentils and add to the vegetable mixture. Simmer for 10 minutes. Serve.

COOKING TIP: Rinse the lentils in a strainer to remove any sediment and check for any small rocks or debris.

PER SERVING: Calories: 454; Total fat: 17g; Protein: 22g; Carbohydrates: 72g; Fiber: 23g; Sugar: 15g; Sodium: 151mg

MUSHROOM AND PEA RISOTTO

GLUTEN-FREE, VEGAN

SERVES 2 TO 4 / PREP TIME: 10 MINUTES / COOK TIME: 30 MINUTES

Arborio rice is a short-grain rice very high in starch, which when cooked slowly with plenty of liquid results in a rich creaminess. Cooking risotto is touted as being complicated, but the method is rather simple; it just takes patience and a lot of stirring. Variations like this recipe are referred to as "risotto ai funghi," or risotto with mushrooms.

4 cups low-sodium vegetable stock

3 tablespoons olive oil, divided

1 tablespoon minced garlic

4 ounces cremini mushrooms, cleaned

4 ounces shiitake mushrooms, cleaned

1 cup frozen peas, thawed

1 cup arborio rice

1. In a medium pot, over medium-high heat, bring the vegetable stock to a boil, reduce the heat to low, and cover. Set aside.

2. In a medium pot, heat 2 tablespoons of olive oil over medium heat until shimmering.

3. Add the garlic, mushrooms, and peas to the olive oil and sauté for 5 minutes. Transfer the vegetables to a bowl.

4. In the same (medium) pot, heat the remaining 1 tablespoon of olive oil over medium heat until shimmering. Add the rice and coat with the oil for 1 minute.

5. Using a ladle, add ½ cup of the warm vegetable stock, bring to a simmer over medium heat, and stir constantly until liquid is absorbed.

6. Continue adding ½ cup of vegetable stock at a time, simmering, and waiting for liquid to be absorbed, until all the vegetable stock has been used. This will take a total of 15 to 20 minutes.

7. Remove the rice from the heat and stir in the vegetables.

8. Serve while hot.

COOKING TIP: Do not rinse the rice before cooking because the starch that makes the risotto creamy will be washed away.

PER SERVING: Calories: 638; Total fat: 21g; Protein: 14g; Carbohydrates: 98g; Fiber: 6g; Sugar: 9g; Sodium: 237mg

OKRA AND DIRTY RICE GUMBO

GLUTEN-FREE, VEGAN

SERVES 4 / PREP TIME: 10 MINUTES / COOK TIME: 1 HOUR

Gumbo is a classic Creole dish that typically features shellfish, poultry, or sausage. This vegan preparation does not skimp on the traditional flavors. This recipe has a twist, crossing gumbo with dirty rice, a Cajun dish that is usually made with chicken liver or ground beef, which gives the rice a "dirty" color. This recipe features black beans to give a meaty texture and the "dirty" flair.

2 tablespoons olive oil

1 green bell pepper, minced

1 small onion, minced

4 celery stalks, minced

10 okra pods, diced

1 (15-ounce) can no-salt-added black beans, drained and rinsed

1 cup brown rice

3 tablespoons minced garlic

1 teaspoon dried thyme

½ teaspoon freshly ground black pepper

32 ounces low-sodium vegetable stock

Hot sauce, for serving

1. In a large stockpot, heat the olive oil on medium heat until it shimmers.

2. Sauté the bell pepper, onion, celery, and okra for 5 to 10 minutes, until they begin to soften.

3. Add the beans, rice, garlic, thyme, pepper, and vegetable stock. Cover and cook on high for 45 minutes.

4. Serve with hot sauce of your choice.

COOKING TIP: You can serve the gumbo as soon as the rice is tender, but stewing the ingredients together for longer really allows the flavors to marry.

PER SERVING: Calories: 369; Total fat: 9g; Protein: 12g; Carbohydrates: 63g; Fiber: 9g; Sugar: 5g; Sodium: 114mg

PINE NUT AND SPINACH PENNE

CONTAINS NUTS, 30 MINUTES, VEGAN
SERVES 4 / PREP TIME: 10 MINUTES / COOK TIME: 15 MINUTES

Pine nuts are the seeds of pine cones. Crunchy yet tender, with a sweet buttery flavor and texture, pine nuts are high in omega-6 fatty acids, monounsaturated (healthy) fats, and vitamin E, which is a natural inflammatory agent. They are also high in manganese, an important nutrient in building antioxidants in the body to fight free radicals.

4 cups water

8 ounces whole-wheat penne

2 tablespoons olive oil

¼ cup pine nuts

1 tablespoon minced garlic

8 cups baby spinach

Red pepper flakes

1. In a large pot, bring the water to a boil.

2. Boil the pasta for 10 to 12 minutes, until tender. Drain.

3. In a large and deep sauté pan or skillet, heat the olive oil over medium heat until shimmering.

4. Toast the pine nuts in the pan for 1 to 2 minutes, stirring frequently.

5. Add the cooked pasta to the pine nuts and stir in the minced garlic and spinach. Cook together until the spinach starts to wilt, 1 to 2 minutes.

6. Season with red pepper flakes and serve.

COOKING TIP: You can make this a cold pasta salad by building a spinach salad, topped with leftover penne and pine nuts, with a simple dressing of olive oil, garlic, and red pepper flakes.

PER SERVING: Calories: 314; Total fat: 14g; Protein: 9g; Carbohydrates: 46g; Fiber: 8g; Sugar: 2g; Sodium: 48mg

RATATOUILLE

GLUTEN-FREE, ONE-POT, VEGAN
SERVES 4 / PREP TIME: 20 MINUTES / COOK TIME: 1 HOUR

Ratatouille is a stewed vegetable dish from the Provence region of France featuring a wide variety of vegetables, depending on the cook. Squash, peppers, eggplant, tomato, and onion are common ingredients.

Nonstick cooking spray

1 orange bell pepper

1 small yellow onion

1 eggplant

1 yellow squash

4 large hothouse tomatoes

1 (15-ounce) can no-salt-added tomato sauce

1 teaspoon minced garlic

½ teaspoon dried basil

½ teaspoon dried thyme

½ teaspoon freshly ground black pepper

1. Preheat the oven to 350°F.

2. Coat the bottom and sides of a 9-inch cake pan with nonstick spray.

3. Using a mandoline or sharp knife, slice ⅛-inch round slices of the bell pepper, onion, eggplant, squash, and tomatoes. This step is much easier and faster if you have a mandoline.

4. In a small bowl, mix the tomato sauce, garlic, basil, thyme, and black pepper. Pour into the cake pan.

5. Working from the outside in, stack slices of each vegetable, in alternating patterns, until you have filled the pan with spirals of rainbow-colored vegetables.

6. Cover the pan with aluminum foil and roast for 45 minutes.

7. Remove the foil and roast for 15 additional minutes.

8. Serve with a spoonful of the pan sauce on top.

COOKING TIP: This is a great recipe to use produce that is past peak freshness, which makes it perfect for reducing food waste.

PER SERVING: Calories: 173; Total fat: 8g; Protein: 4g; Carbohydrates: 25g; Fiber: 8g; Sugar: 14g; Sodium: 57mg

RED BEANS AND RICE

GLUTEN-FREE, SLOW COOKER, VEGAN
SERVES 4 / PREP TIME: 10 MINUTES (PLUS SOAKING OVERNIGHT) / COOK TIME: 6 HOURS

Red beans and rice is a classic Creole dish. The base of this staple is the "holy trinity" of Southern cooking: bell pepper, onion, and celery. Adding garlic to this trinity is called "adding the pope."

FOR THE RED BEANS

1 pound dried red beans

6 cups water

1 green bell pepper, minced

1 small onion, minced

4 celery stalks, minced

3 tablespoons minced garlic

1 teaspoon freshly ground black pepper

1 teaspoon dried sage

1 teaspoon dried thyme

½ teaspoon cayenne pepper

3 bay leaves

32 ounces low-sodium vegetable stock

FOR THE RICE

2 cups water

1 cup brown rice

FOR THE SLURRY

3 tablespoons cornstarch

¼ cup water

1. In a large bowl, soak the beans in water overnight. Drain and rinse the beans.

2. In a slow cooker, combine the beans, bell pepper, onion, celery, garlic, black pepper, sage, thyme, cayenne pepper, bay leaves, and vegetable stock. Cover and cook on high for 6 hours.

3. With 1 hour remaining of cooking, in a medium pot, boil the water for the rice.

4. Add the rice to the boiling water, reduce the heat to low, and cover. Cook for 45 minutes.

5. In a small bowl, make a slurry by whisking the cornstarch into the water. Pour the slurry into the slow cooker and stir thoroughly to thicken the red bean mixture.

6. Remove the bay leaves (though finding a bay leaf in your food is said to bring good luck). Serve over a bed of rice.

VARIATION TIP: Traditional red beans and rice includes andouille sausage. This recipe can be made to include poultry and still fit into the MIND Diet. Simply use ground chicken or turkey, and season it with paprika, garlic, pepper, onion, cayenne pepper, oregano, and thyme.

PER SERVING: Calories: 426; Total fat: 1g; Protein: 27g; Carbohydrates: 121g; Fiber: 56g; Sugar: 6g; Sodium: 194mg

RED PEPPER PASTA

VEGAN

SERVES 4 / PREP TIME: 10 MINUTES / COOK TIME: 1 HOUR

Red bell peppers are a fresh, sweet, and mildly spicy vegetable that add a new twist to pasta sauce. They are high in free radical–fighting antioxidants. Puréeing the pepper creates a light-colored foam that lightens the tomato sauce and adds creaminess to this dish, which is certain to become a new favorite.

1 red bell pepper, halved and seeded

4 cups water

8 ounces whole-wheat linguine

1 (15-ounce) can no-salt-added tomato sauce

1 teaspoon onion powder

1 teaspoon garlic powder

1 teaspoon Italian seasoning

½ teaspoon cayenne pepper

¼ cup minced fresh parsley

1. Preheat the oven to 400°F.

2. On a foil-lined baking sheet, roast the pepper halves, skin-side up, for 45 minutes. Charring on the outside of the pepper is normal.

3. During the last 15 minutes of roasting, in a large pot, begin boiling the water.

4. Boil the pasta for 10 to 12 minutes, until tender. Drain.

5. In a blender, purée the roasted red bell pepper, tomato sauce, onion powder, garlic powder, Italian seasoning, and cayenne pepper on high for 10 to 20 seconds.

6. Add the sauce to the pasta and mix thoroughly.

7. Serve with fresh parsley sprinkled on top.

COOKING TIP: You can roast bell peppers whole and then chill in an ice bath until they are cool enough to handle to remove the core and the seeds. You can also peel the skin off the roasted peppers if you prefer.

VARIATION TIP: Make this recipe gluten-free by substituting your favorite gluten-free noodles.

PER SERVING: Calories: 221; Total fat: 2g; Protein: 7g; Carbohydrates: 50g; Fiber: 9g; Sugar: 4g; Sodium: 38mg

TABBOULEH

30 MINUTES, VEGAN
SERVES 2 TO 4 / PREP TIME: 5 MINUTES / COOK TIME: 15 MINUTES

Tabbouleh is a vegetarian dish from the Levantine region. It is typically served as a side dish but is a delicious vegan entrée on the MIND diet. It consists of fresh herbs, whole grains, and vegetables.

1 cup water

1 cup bulgur

2 bunches parsley

1 bunch mint

2 English cucumbers

1 large hothouse tomato

¼ cup olive oil

¼ cup lemon juice

1 teaspoon freshly ground black pepper

1. In a microwave-safe bowl, microwave the water for 2 minutes, or until boiling.

2. Add the bulgur to the water and let sit for 7 to 15 minutes, until all water is absorbed and the grains are tender.

3. While the bulgur is soaking, finely chop the parsley and mint leaves. Set aside in a large bowl.

4. Dice the cucumbers and the tomato and add them to the bowl.

5. Add the olive oil, lemon juice, and black pepper to the bowl and stir.

6. Combine the bulgur with the vegetables. Mix thoroughly.

COOKING TIP: The bulgur most commonly found in stores will need to be soaked for 7 to 15 minutes. Coarser ground bulgur is harder to find but can be used without soaking.

VARIATION TIP: Add chickpeas to this recipe for the added benefit of plant-based protein.

PER SERVING: Calories: 598; Total fat: 29g; Protein: 16g; Carbohydrates: 78g; Fiber: 19g; Sugar: 11g; Sodium: 92mg

TOFU STIR-FRY

VEGAN

SERVES 2 TO 4 / PREP TIME: 1 HOUR / COOK TIME: 40 MINUTES

Stir-frying allows for maximum levels of fresh flavor and texture of the vegetables, with minimal oil needed. The technique used in this recipe is called "chao," which is a method similar to sautéing. Serve over your favorite noodles or rice.

FOR THE TOFU
14 ounces extra-firm tofu

FOR THE MARINADE
1 tablespoon low-sodium soy sauce

1 tablespoon agave syrup

1 tablespoon lemon juice

1 tablespoon minced garlic

½ teaspoon ground ginger

FOR THE STIR-FRY
2 tablespoons olive oil

1 large head of broccoli, chopped

2 carrots, sliced

1 red bell pepper, sliced

1 cup sugar snap peas

1 (8-ounce) can water chestnuts, drained

1. Line a plate with several paper towels. Remove the tofu block from the package and place it on the paper towels.

2. Add additional paper towels on top of the tofu block and place a cutting board on top of the paper towels.

3. Weigh the cutting board down with a heavy book, a pot, or several cans.

4. Leave the tofu to drain for at least 30 minutes.

5. Cut the tofu into 1-inch cubes.

6. In a large bowl, whisk together the marinade of soy sauce, agave syrup, lemon juice, garlic, and ginger.

7. Marinate the tofu for 30 minutes.

8. In a large and deep sauté pan or skillet or a wok, heat the olive oil on medium heat until shimmering.

9. Stir-fry the broccoli and carrots for 5 minutes.

10. Add the bell pepper, peas, water chestnuts, and tofu and stir-fry for 5 more minutes. Serve.

SUBSTITUTION TIP: Substitute tamari for the soy sauce to make this dish gluten-free.

PER SERVING: Calories: 550; Total fat: 25g; Protein: 34g; Carbohydrates: 59g; Fiber: 18g; Sugar: 21g; Sodium: 484mg

ZOODLES

GLUTEN-FREE, 30 MINUTES, VEGAN
SERVES 2 TO 4 / PREP TIME: 10 MINUTES / COOK TIME: 10 MINUTES

Zucchini noodles have grown in popularity for gluten-free diets and for people who love pasta but believe they need to reduce their carbohydrates. Zoodles are great not only as a pasta substitute, but as a dish all on their own. The bright and fresh green flavor of zucchini is enhanced by being sautéed in olive oil and pepper, and zoodles make the perfect side dish or base for a heartier meal.

¼ cup olive oil

4 large zucchini, spiralized

½ teaspoon freshly ground black pepper

1. In a medium sauté pan or skillet, heat the olive oil on medium heat until shimmering.

2. Sauté the zucchini noodles and pepper for 6 to 8 minutes. Remove the zoodles from the heat if they are releasing a lot of moisture into the pan; this will prevent them from becoming soggy. Serve.

COOKING TIP: You can spiralize noodles from zucchini using a spiralizer, a mandoline, or a julienne peeler. A handheld spiralizer is very easy to use, is inexpensive, and can be found at most retailers.

PER SERVING: Calories: 344; Total fat: 29g; Protein: 8g; Carbohydrates: 22g; Fiber: 7g; Sugar: 11g; Sodium: 64mg

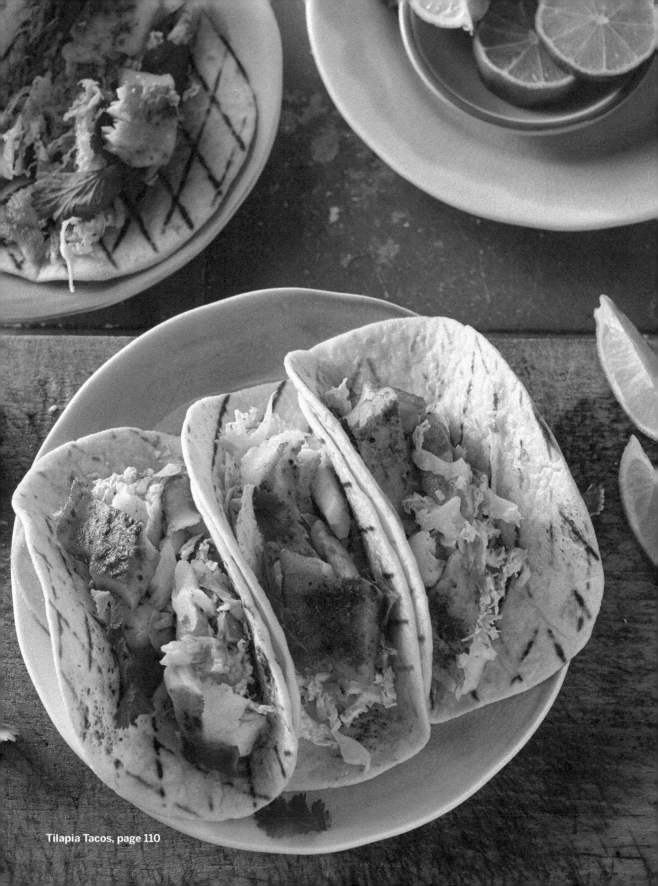

Tilapia Tacos, page 110

SEAFOOD ENTRÉES

Seafood is an important part of the MIND diet, due to its high omega-3 fatty acid content, healthy unsaturated fats, B vitamins, and protein. The variety of recipes in this chapter will have you craving seafood, which is a requirement to eat at least once per week on the MIND diet. These recipes have been carefully curated to teach you a variety of cooking methods and expose you to 15 different varieties of seafood. From sardines to halibut, shrimp to anchovies, there is a seafood dish to satisfy any craving.

Seafood is a wonderful addition to pastas, soups, tacos, and vegetable dishes. If you have not previously been a fan of seafood, these recipes provide the opportunity to branch out and try new flavors. Recipes in this chapter are rich in omega-3 fatty acids, which have been shown to help reduce inflammation in the body and, according to various studies, may be linked to a reduced risk of Alzheimer's disease and a decrease in age-related cognitive decline. Dishes with an especially high amount of omega-3s include Garlic-Broccoli-Anchovy Pasta (page 98), Ladolemono Salmon and Brussels Sprouts (page 100), Smoked Herring and Cabbage (page 107), and Tilapia Tacos (page 110).

ALLERGY NOTE: If you are allergic to shellfish, feel free to use your favorite fish instead in the Cioppino (page 96), Honey-Garlic Shrimp with "Burnt" Broccoli (page 99), and Scallop Linguine (page 106) recipes.

SODIUM AND MERCURY

Most grocery chains stock a wide variety of whole fish, fish fillets, and shellfish that may have been frozen for transport to ensure food safety. You can also find canned seafood varieties, which are convenient and tasty options on the MIND diet. Keep in mind, however, that most canned seafood is packed in salted water or some sort of plant oil. But while these contain higher levels of sodium, they are still rich sources of protein and omega-3 fatty acids. Draining the liquid from the can reduces the amount of added salt.

Mercury is a concern for many when including seafood in their diet. It is safe to eat 12 ounces of lower-mercury fish per week, and all the recipes in this chapter fit within those parameters. Low-mercury fish include canned light tuna, shrimp, catfish, tilapia, sardines, trout, salmon, and pollock. High-mercury fish include shark, tilefish, swordfish, and king mackerel. The mercury content is higher because these fish eat more mercury-containing algae than smaller fish, and also eat smaller fish that contain mercury.

CATFISH AMANDINE

CONTAINS NUTS, GLUTEN-FREE, 30 MINUTES
SERVES 4 / PREP TIME: 10 MINUTES / COOK TIME: 20 MINUTES

Amandine is a culinary preparation that simply means "with almonds." Typically, as in this recipe, the almonds are sliced and toasted in oil and spices. Almonds are a beautiful crunchy addition to both the catfish and green beans, adding additional protein, fiber, healthy fat, and vitamin E.

⅓ cup cornstarch

1 teaspoon paprika

2 tablespoons olive oil, divided

1 tablespoon minced garlic

1 pound green beans

¼ cup sliced unsalted almonds

2 (8-ounce) catfish fillets, skinless

½ lemon

1. On a large plate, prepare the cornstarch dredge by mixing the cornstarch with the paprika. Set aside.

2. In a medium sauté pan or skillet, heat 1 tablespoon of olive oil over medium heat until shimmering.

3. Sauté the garlic, green beans, and almonds for 10 minutes.

4. While the green beans are sautéing, dredge the catfish in the cornstarch and paprika mixture.

5. Remove the green beans and almonds from the pan and set aside.

6. Add the remaining 1 tablespoon of olive oil to the pan and heat over medium heat until shimmering. Add the catfish fillets to the pan.

7. Fry the catfish for 5 minutes, flip, and fry the other side for 5 minutes, or until golden brown.

8. Serve with fresh-squeezed lemon juice.

SUBSTITUTION TIP: If you cannot find catfish, tilapia is the best substitute.

PER SERVING: Calories: 336; Total fat: 14g; Protein: 34g; Carbohydrates: 22g; Fiber: 6g; Sugar: 4g; Sodium: 87mg

CIOPPINO

GLUTEN-FREE, ONE-POT
SERVES 4 / PREP TIME: 20 MINUTES / COOK TIME: 45 MINUTES

While cioppino has Italian influences, it actually comes from San Francisco, California. Traditionally, it is made from the fresh catches of the day. This recipe includes staples of firm white fish, shrimp, and clams, but any seafood is delicious in this seafood stew. Clams and mussels are very high in omega-3 fatty acids, as is cod. Shrimp also contain omega-3 fatty acids, as well as antioxidants, which make them a great food on the MIND diet.

2 tablespoons olive oil

1 yellow onion, diced

1 fennel bulb, diced

3 tablespoons minced garlic

32 ounces low-sodium vegetable stock

1 (15-ounce) can no-salt-added crushed tomatoes

2 cups dry white wine

2 tablespoons dried oregano

½ pound cod

½ pound large shrimp

1 pound clams or mussels

1 lemon, halved

1. In a large pot, over medium heat, heat the olive oil until shimmering.

2. Sauté the onion, fennel, and garlic for 10 minutes.

3. Add the vegetable stock, crushed tomatoes, wine, and oregano to the pot.

4. Bring the pot to a boil, reduce the heat to medium, cover, and cook for 30 minutes.

5. While the broth and vegetables are cooking, cut the cod into 2-inch cubes, peel and devein the shrimp, and rinse the clams.

6. Reduce the heat to medium-low, add the seafood to the broth and vegetable mixture, and simmer for 10 minutes.

7. Squeeze the lemon juice into the cioppino and serve.

COOKING TIP: Clams or mussels should be completely closed prior to cooking; throw away any that have opened or are cracked. After cooking, discard any clams or mussels that did not open.

PER SERVING: Calories: 443; Total fat: 10g; Protein: 42g; Carbohydrates: 27g; Fiber: 6g; Sugar: 10g; Sodium: 286mg

COD CHOWDER

GLUTEN-FREE, ONE-POT

SERVES 2 TO 4 / PREP TIME: 10 MINUTES / COOK TIME: 30 MINUTES

Cod is a less oily fish than salmon or sardines but contains a good amount of omega-3 fatty acids. It has a mild flavor and a meaty texture. Cod-liver oil is sold in capsule form as an omega-3 fatty acid supplement because the liver has higher fat content than the fish itself. Many other fish oil supplements are derived from mackerel, herring, anchovies, or tuna.

2 tablespoons olive oil

1 large leek, diced

2 celery stalks, diced

½ yellow onion, diced

4 cups low-sodium vegetable stock

1 tablespoon white wine vinegar

¼ teaspoon freshly ground black pepper

½ pound new potatoes, diced

1 (15-ounce) can no-salt-added cannellini beans, drained and rinsed

2 (4-ounce) cod fillets, cubed

1 head baby bok choy, chopped

1. In a large pot, over medium heat, heat the olive oil until shimmering.

2. Sauté the leek, celery, and onion for 10 minutes.

3. Add the vegetable stock, vinegar, pepper, potatoes, and beans to the pot and simmer for 10 minutes.

4. Add the cod and bok choy and simmer for 5 minutes, or until the fish is opaque and cooked through.

SUBSTITUTION TIP: Any leafy green, such as spinach, kale, chard, collard greens, or cabbage, would work well in this recipe.

PER SERVING: Calories: 294; Total fat: 9g; Protein: 21g; Carbohydrates: 33g; Fiber: 9g; Sugar: 3g; Sodium: 269mg

GARLIC-BROCCOLI-ANCHOVY PASTA

CONTAINS NUTS, 30 MINUTES

SERVES 4 / PREP TIME: 5 MINUTES / COOK TIME: 15 MINUTES

Anchovies are oily saltwater fish high in omega-3 fatty acids. They are also rich in niacin, a B vitamin with strong cardiovascular benefits, vitamins A and E, potassium, calcium, and the antioxidant-rich mineral selenium. These tiny fish fillets are a perfect food for the MIND diet and are packed with flavor.

6 cups water

8 ounces whole-wheat spaghetti

2 cups broccoli florets

2 tablespoons olive oil

2 tablespoons minced garlic

2 (2-ounce) cans anchovy fillets, oil reserved

¼ cup pine nuts

¼ cup chopped fresh parsley

1. In a large pot, bring the water to a boil.

2. Boil the pasta for 10 to 12 minutes, until tender.

3. While the pasta is cooking, in a large and deep sauté pan or skillet, over medium heat, combine the olive oil, minced garlic, anchovies, and pine nuts.

4. Cook for 5 minutes, creating the sauce.

5. During the last 5 minutes of cooking the pasta, add the broccoli florets to the pot to cook. Drain.

6. Add the pasta and broccoli to the pan sauce and toss until evenly coated.

7. Serve topped with the fresh parsley.

VARIATION TIP: Red pepper flakes make a spicy addition to this dish, if you prefer things on the hotter side.

PER SERVING: Calories: 375; Total fat: 16g; Protein: 12g; Carbohydrates: 46g; Fiber: 7g; Sugar: 3g; Sodium: 913mg

HONEY-GARLIC SHRIMP WITH "BURNT" BROCCOLI

GLUTEN-FREE

SERVES 2 TO 4 / PREP TIME: 5 MINUTES / COOK TIME: 30 MINUTES

"Burnt" broccoli is a different way of preparing a vegetable that is typically steamed or eaten raw. Roasting the broccoli in the oven until the florets are slightly charred gives the broccoli a nutty flavor that pairs deliciously with the sweet caramelized shrimp in this dish.

2 large heads broccoli

1 tablespoon olive oil

Freshly ground black pepper

2 cups water

1 cup brown rice

1 pound large shrimp, peeled and deveined

1 teaspoon minced garlic

2 tablespoons honey

¼ teaspoon cayenne pepper (optional)

1. Preheat the oven to 400°F.

2. Cut the broccoli into bite-size pieces, drizzle with the olive oil, and season with pepper.

3. Spread the broccoli in a single layer on a foil-covered baking sheet and roast for 30 minutes, checking to prevent burning.

4. While the broccoli is roasting, in a large pot, bring the water to a boil over high heat. Add the rice to the boiling water, reduce the heat to low, and cover. Cook for 15 to 20 minutes, until all the water is absorbed.

5. Coat the shrimp in the garlic, honey, and cayenne pepper (if using).

6. In a large sauté pan or skillet, sauté the shrimp until they are pink, about 5 minutes. The garlic-and-honey mixture should caramelize the exterior of the shrimp.

7. Serve the shrimp and the broccoli over a bed of rice.

INGREDIENT TIP: If you are not comfortable cooking raw shrimp, you can purchase precooked shrimp at the seafood counter at the grocery store. Reheating will not overcook the shrimp or make them rubbery.

PER SERVING: Calories: 686; Total fat: 14g; Protein: 74g; Carbohydrates: 87g; Fiber: 20g; Sugar: 28g; Sodium: 2,063mg

LADOLEMONO SALMON AND BRUSSELS SPROUTS

GLUTEN-FREE, 30 MINUTES

SERVES 2 TO 4 / PREP TIME: 15 MINUTES / COOK TIME: 15 MINUTES

Brussels sprouts are nutrient-bomb tiny cabbages that pack a big punch. Brussels sprouts are high in vitamin K and vitamin C, and have modest amounts of vitamin A, folate, and manganese. Roasting Brussels sprouts in the oven gives them a sweetness and nuttiness, along with a crunch, that defy anyone who grew up hating Brussels sprouts. The ladolemono sauce is a classic Mediterranean lemon-mustard-dill sauce that complements the salmon and Brussels sprouts perfectly.

FOR THE LADOLEMONO SAUCE

¼ cup lemon juice

¼ cup olive oil

2 tablespoons stone-ground mustard

¼ teaspoon freshly ground black pepper

½ teaspoon dried oregano

2 tablespoons chopped fresh parsley

½ teaspoon chopped fresh dill

2 teaspoons minced garlic

FOR THE SALMON

20 large Brussels sprouts

2 (4-ounce) salmon fillets, skinless

1. Preheat the oven to 400°F.

2. Prepare the ladolemono sauce by whisking together the lemon juice, olive oil, mustard, pepper, oregano, parsley, dill, and garlic in a small bowl. Set aside 2 tablespoons of the sauce to drizzle over the salmon.

3. Cut the stems from the Brussels sprouts and cut each in half.

4. Peel the leaves of each Brussels sprout from the heart.

5. Mix the ladolemono with the Brussels sprouts leaves and hearts.

6. Roast the Brussels sprouts on a parchment paper–lined baking sheet for 15 minutes, checking to prevent burning.

7. Make a foil boat for the salmon by folding up the edges of a piece of foil to create walls.

8. On the same baking sheet, roast the salmon in the foil boat for 15 minutes, until the fish is opaque and flakes easily with a fork.

9. Drizzle the reserved ladolemono sauce on the salmon and serve along with the Brussels sprouts.

INGREDIENT TIP: You can purchase salmon with the skin on or off. If you purchase skin-on salmon, you can either cut it off with a fillet knife or cook it with the skin on. If your salmon skin still has scales on it, you can descale it by scraping it with a sharp knife against the grain of the scales. You can tell the scales are coming off when the skin has a "fishnet" look to it.

PER SERVING: Calories: 475; Total fat: 32g; Protein: 30g; Carbohydrates: 21g; Fiber: 8g; Sugar: 5g; Sodium: 246mg

ONE-PAN HALIBUT

GLUTEN-FREE, ONE-POT, 30 MINUTES
SERVES 4 / PREP TIME: 10 MINUTES / COOK TIME: 20 MINUTES

Halibut are flatfish loved for their white flesh and delicate flavor. They are particularly high in selenium, a trace mineral that is a powerful antioxidant. The high omega-3 fatty acid content of halibut helps reduce inflammation, and the niacin content can help improve blood flow. A fun fact is that halibut can grow to over 600 pounds!

1 tablespoon olive oil

1 cup cherry tomatoes, halved

1 cup fresh or thawed frozen green peas

1 teaspoon minced garlic

4 (4-ounce) halibut fillets, skinless

1 tablespoon chopped fresh dill

¼ teaspoon freshly ground black pepper

1 lemon, halved

1. In a medium sauté pan or skillet over medium heat, heat the olive oil until shimmering.

2. Sauté the tomatoes, peas, and garlic for 10 minutes.

3. While the vegetables are sautéing, season the halibut with the dill and pepper.

4. Move the vegetables to one side of the pan and add the halibut fillets to the pan.

5. Sear the halibut and cook for 5 minutes, flip, and sear the other side and cook for 5 minutes.

6. Serve with fresh-squeezed lemon juice.

SUBSTITUTION TIP: Halibut is a pricier fillet of fish and can be replaced with bass, cod, fluke, or flounder.

PER SERVING: Calories: 238; Total fat: 7g; Protein: 33g; Carbohydrates: 11g; Fiber: 4g; Sugar: 3g; Sodium: 113mg

ROCKFISH-WATERMELON TACOS

GLUTEN-FREE
SERVES 4 / PREP TIME: 10 MINUTES / COOK TIME: 25 MINUTES

Rockfish are also known as red snapper or rock cod, and can live for up to 200 years. They do not produce many young, and are often overfished, which makes them expensive. Rockfish may be low in omega-3 fatty acids, but are rich in selenium and vitamins B_6 and B_{12}, which have strong neurological benefits.

2 (8-ounce) rockfish fillets, skinless

1 teaspoon chili powder

1 teaspoon chipotle chile powder

1 teaspoon ground cumin

1 teaspoon garlic powder

1 small icebox watermelon

½ red onion

1 jalapeño

1 tablespoon lime juice

8 corn tortillas

1. Preheat the oven to 400°F.

2. Pat the rockfish dry and rub with the chili powder, chipotle chile powder, cumin, and garlic powder.

3. On a foil-lined baking sheet, bake the rockfish for 20 to 25 minutes, until it is opaque and flakes with a fork.

4. While the rockfish is cooking, prepare the watermelon salsa. Remove the rind and dice the watermelon, then dice the onion and jalapeño.

5. In a medium bowl, mix the watermelon, onion, and jalapeño with the lime juice and set aside.

6. In a large sauté pan or skillet, on high heat, brown the corn tortillas in batches for 1 minute per side.

7. Build each taco by filling the tortilla with rockfish and garnishing with the watermelon salsa. Serve.

INGREDIENT TIP: A mango salsa or pico de gallo would also be delicious on these tacos in place of the watermelon salsa. The mild and sweet flavor of the rockfish is very versatile.

SUBSTITUTION TIP: Cod is a suitable substitute if you cannot find rockfish.

PER SERVING: Calories: 308; Total fat: 4g; Protein: 32g; Carbohydrates: 38g; Fiber: 5g; Sugar: 11g; Sodium: 126mg

SARDINES WITH ARTICHOKES AND GREENS

GLUTEN-FREE

SERVES 4 / PREP TIME: 10 MINUTES / COOK TIME: 30 MINUTES (PLUS 30 MINUTES TO COOL)

Sardines are an oily fish high in omega-3 fatty acids, calcium, iron, and B vitamins. You can buy sardines that are skinless and boneless, but both the skin and bones are edible, so it is completely up to preference. They make a great snack or an addition to pasta or salad, as in this recipe, because they do not require additional cooking.

2 artichokes

2 cups water

1 tablespoon Dijon mustard

2 tablespoons olive oil

2 tablespoons white wine vinegar

8 cups arugula

4 (4.4-ounce) cans sardines in water, drained

1. On a cutting board, using a sharp serrated knife, cut off the top third of the artichokes, as this portion is inedible. Also cut off the bottom half of the stems.

2. In a large pot, cover the artichokes with water. Cover with a lid.

3. Bring the water to a boil over medium-high heat.

4. Cook for 30 minutes.

5. Drain and set the artichokes aside to cool for 30 minutes.

6. Cut each artichoke in half down the stem.

7. For the dressing, in a large bowl, whisk together the mustard, olive oil, and vinegar.

8. Toss the arugula in the dressing.

9. Serve the sardines on top of the salad and enjoy the tender artichoke leaves on the side.

10. To eat the artichokes, peel a leaf off the stem and use your teeth to scrape the flesh from the leaf. The stem and heart of the artichoke are edible and often the tastiest part.

SUBSTITUTION TIP: Your favorite vinegar can replace the white wine vinegar in the dressing, such as red wine vinegar or sherry vinegar.

INGREDIENT TIP: Sardines are commonly purchased in a can, and come packed in water, oil, or tomato sauce. Taste testing a few varieties may help you find your favorite.

PER SERVING: Calories: 249; Total fat: 16g; Protein: 19g; Carbohydrates: 8g; Fiber: 4g; Sugar: 2g; Sodium: 463mg

SCALLOP LINGUINE

30 MINUTES

SERVES 4 / PREP TIME: 5 MINUTES / COOK TIME: 15 MINUTES

Scallops can be purchased fresh or frozen, but fresh scallops are likely to be found in states bordering the Atlantic Ocean. Scallops are high in omega-3 fatty acids, numerous vitamins, and important trace minerals such as selenium and zinc.

4 cups water

8 ounces whole-wheat linguine

2 tablespoons olive oil, divided

2 tablespoons lemon juice

¼ teaspoon freshly ground black pepper

¼ teaspoon red pepper flakes (optional)

1 pound scallops, blotted dry

1. In a large pot, bring the water to a boil.

2. Boil the pasta for 10 to 12 minutes, until tender. Drain.

3. Add 1 tablespoon of olive oil, the lemon juice, black pepper, and red pepper flakes (if using) to the pasta, creating the sauce.

4. In a small sauté pan or skillet, heat the remaining 1 tablespoon of olive oil over medium heat until shimmering.

5. Sear the scallops in a single layer for 90 seconds. Flip the scallops and sear the other side for 90 seconds. The scallops are done when they turn opaque.

6. Serve the pasta topped with the scallops.

VARIATION TIP: Make this recipe gluten-free by substituting your favorite gluten-free noodles.

PER SERVING: Calories: 342; Total fat: 10g; Protein: 25g; Carbohydrates: 44g; Fiber: 6g; Sugar: <1g; Sodium: 184mg

SMOKED HERRING AND CABBAGE

GLUTEN-FREE

SERVES 2 TO 4 / PREP TIME: 10 MINUTES / COOK TIME: 30 MINUTES

Herring are saltwater fish, high in omega-3 fatty acids. They are often prepared using salt curing, smoking, or pickling, which makes them high in sodium. This recipe uses boiling and rinsing to remove some of the sodium.

3 cups water

12 ounces smoked herring

2 tablespoons olive oil

2 tablespoons minced garlic

2 scallions, green parts only, chopped

1 cup grape tomatoes, halved

½ head cabbage, shredded

Coarsely ground black pepper

1. In a medium pot, bring the water to a boil over high heat. Add the smoked herring and boil for 10 minutes.

2. Using a mesh strainer or colander, rinse the herring under cool running water for 30 seconds. Transfer the herring to paper towels to drain for 10 minutes.

3. Remove the skin and debone if necessary. Flake the fish apart using 2 forks or your fingers.

4. In a large and deep sauté pan or skillet, heat the olive oil on medium heat until it shimmers.

5. Sauté the garlic, scallions, and tomatoes for 10 minutes.

6. Add the herring and cabbage and sauté, covered, for 10 minutes to allow the cabbage to wilt.

7. Season with coarsely ground pepper and serve.

COOKING TIP: Smoked herring can be purchased as whole fish from certain retailers, or as boneless fillets in cans.

SUBSTITUTION TIP: You can replace the herring with mackerel or catfish. If using one of these alternative fish, skip steps 1 through 3.

PER SERVING: Calories: 628; Total fat: 48g; Protein: 40g; Carbohydrates: 20g; Fiber: 7g; Sugar: 9g; Sodium: 889mg

SPICY TROUT

GLUTEN-FREE, ONE-POT, 30 MINUTES
SERVES 4 / PREP TIME: 15 MINUTES / COOK TIME: 10 MINUTES

This recipe has only four simple ingredients, but when it is prepared correctly, it is irresistible. Trout are freshwater fish high in omega-3 fatty acids, B vitamins, potassium, and phosphorus. They have a light pink flesh with many flavor similarities to salmon. Fish skin is a great source of omega-3 fatty acids and is a crispy treat.

4 whole brook trout, butterflied and scaled

2 tablespoons olive oil

2 red chiles, seeded and sliced

1 lemon, halved

1. Thoroughly pat the trout dry.

2. In a large sauté pan or skillet, heat the olive oil on medium heat until it shimmers.

3. Fry the trout and chiles for 5 minutes. Flip the trout and fry the other side for 5 minutes, or until golden brown. The fish will turn opaque and easily flake with a fork.

4. Serve with fresh-squeezed lemon juice on top.

COOKING TIP: Trout skin is perfectly fine to eat. You can scale it by scraping it with a sharp knife against the grain of the scales. You can tell the scales are coming off when the skin has a "fishnet" look to it.

SUBSTITUTION TIP: Rainbow trout fillets would also work well in this recipe.

PER SERVING: Calories: 256; Total fat: 19g; Protein: 21g; Carbohydrates: 5g; Fiber: 2g; Sugar: 1g; Sodium: 3mg

SWEET PEPPER MACKEREL

GLUTEN-FREE, 30 MINUTES
SERVES 4 / PREP TIME: 10 MINUTES / COOK TIME: 15 MINUTES

Mackerel are saltwater fish that have a milder taste than salmon but are consumed much less often because they are harder to find inland. They are an oily fish high in omega-3 fatty acids, perfect on the MIND diet (if you can find them, though salmon makes a suitable substitute). They take on the flavor of what they are cooked with, allowing the sweet peppers to shine.

FOR THE MACKEREL

2 tablespoons olive oil

2 cups sweet cherry peppers, sliced

2 (8-ounce) mackerel fillets

½ teaspoon sweet paprika

FOR THE DRESSING

2 tablespoons olive oil

1 tablespoon white wine vinegar

¼ teaspoon freshly ground black pepper

¼ teaspoon sweet paprika

1. In a medium sauté pan or skillet, heat 2 tablespoons of olive oil over medium heat until shimmering.

2. Sauté the sweet cherry peppers for 5 minutes.

3. While the peppers are sautéing, season the mackerel with the sweet paprika.

4. Add the mackerel to the pan and sear for 5 minutes, flip, and sear the other side for 5 minutes.

5. While the mackerel is cooking, in a small bowl create the dressing by whisking together the olive oil, vinegar, pepper, and sweet paprika.

6. Serve the mackerel drizzled with the dressing.

SUBSTITUTION TIP: If you cannot find sweet cherry peppers, red, orange, or yellow bell peppers work well in this dish.

PER SERVING: Calories: 434; Total fat: 35g; Protein: 28g; Carbohydrates: 2g; Fiber: 1g; Sugar: <1g; Sodium: 434mg

TILAPIA TACOS

GLUTEN-FREE, 30 MINUTES
SERVES 4 / PREP TIME: 15 MINUTES / COOK TIME: 15 MINUTES

Tilapia are freshwater white fish with a delicate flavor and tender fillets. Tilapia is a perfect fish for people who dislike "fishy-tasting" fish. Tilapia is a less fatty fish that contains few omega-3 fatty acids per serving, but it is still a source of omega fatty acids and can be included in a varied MIND diet. Tilapia is also very affordable, as seafood can be expensive for people who live inland.

1 tablespoon olive oil

2 (8-ounce) tilapia fillets

1 teaspoon dried oregano

⅛ teaspoon chili powder

⅛ teaspoon garlic powder

⅛ teaspoon onion powder

⅛ teaspoon cayenne pepper (optional)

1 cup plain coleslaw mix (or shredded cabbage)

1 small Roma tomato, diced

1 tablespoon lime juice

8 corn tortillas

1. In a medium sauté pan or skillet, heat the olive oil over medium heat until shimmering.

2. Coat the tilapia fillets with the oregano, chili powder, garlic powder, onion powder, and cayenne pepper (if using).

3. Cook the tilapia for 4 to 5 minutes per side, until the fish flakes with a fork and is opaque inside.

4. While the tilapia is cooking, in a medium bowl, mix the coleslaw, tomato, and lime juice. Set aside.

5. Remove the tilapia from the pan and allow to rest while you heat the tortillas.

6. Wipe the pan with a paper towel. Working in batches, brown the corn tortillas over high heat for 1 minute per side.

7. Build each taco by filling the corn tortillas with tilapia and topping with the garnish. Serve.

INGREDIENT TIP: These tasty tacos can be topped with shredded lettuce, mixed spring greens, or baby spinach in place of the coleslaw. You can make a pico de gallo with Roma tomato, finely diced onion, and jalapeño to top your tacos. The guacamole and salsa from chapter 3 (page 30) would make a perfect addition.

PER SERVING: Calories: 266; Total fat: 7g; Protein: 27g; Carbohydrates: 26g; Fiber: 4g; Sugar: 2g; Sodium: 88mg

TUNA VEGETABLE WRAP

30 MINUTES

SERVES 4 / PREP TIME: 5 MINUTES

Tuna is an excellent source of lean protein and omega-3 fatty acids, all in a convenient and shelf-stable can. The potassium in tuna enhances the omega-3 fatty acids' already powerful anti-inflammatory properties. Canned tuna is a pantry staple and goes well with different flavors and vegetables.

2 (5-ounce) cans chunk light tuna, drained

2 tablespoons olive oil

1 tablespoon lemon juice

1 tablespoon chopped fresh basil

1 carrot, grated

1 zucchini, grated

4 whole-wheat tortillas

1 cup baby spinach

1. In a large bowl, combine the tuna, olive oil, lemon juice, basil, carrot, and zucchini. Mix until all the ingredients are evenly combined.

2. On each tortilla, spoon ¼ cup of spinach and one-fourth of the tuna salad.

3. Make a wrap by rolling up the ingredients in the tortilla. Serve.

INGREDIENT TIP: Chunk light tuna is preferable to chunk white albacore tuna because of its lower mercury content. Light tuna comes from skipjack tuna, which are smaller fish than the large albacore tuna. The larger the fish, the higher the mercury content. It is safe to consume 12 ounces of chunk light tuna per week. Select tuna packed in water or olive oil and drain off the liquid before serving to reduce the sodium.

PER SERVING: Calories: 257; Total fat: 11g; Protein: 18g; Carbohydrates: 26g; Fiber: 4g; Sugar: 4g; Sodium: 482mg

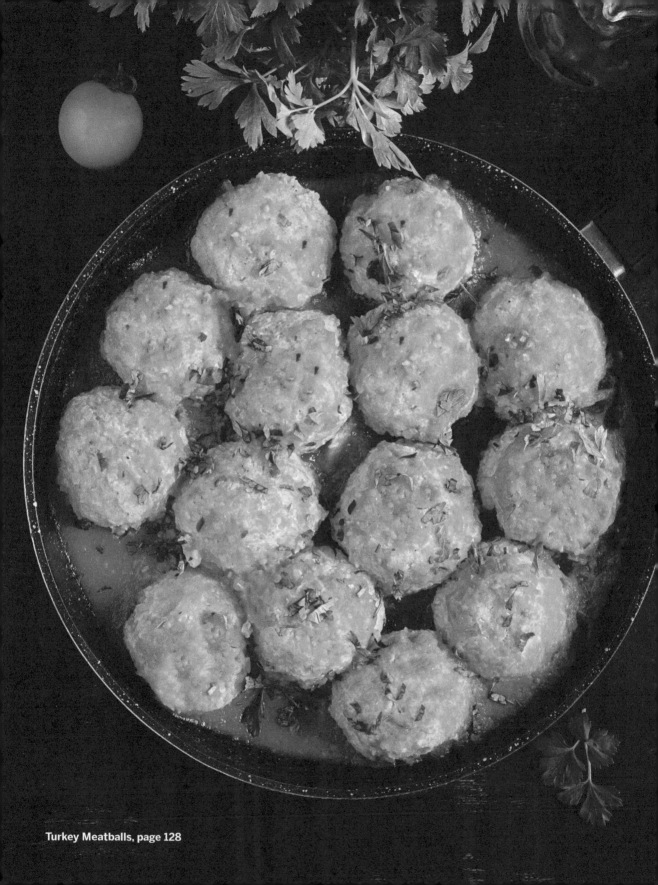

Turkey Meatballs, page 128

CHAPTER EIGHT

POULTRY ENTRÉES

oultry (such as chicken and turkey) meat is an excellent source of low-saturated-fat protein (especially when eaten without the skin) and B vitamins, which contribute to healthy body and brain function. Saturated fat is responsible for cholesterol buildup in the arteries, which increases the risk for heart attack, stroke, and the development of Alzheimer's disease and dementia. Eating a diet lower in saturated fat and higher in unsaturated fat has been linked by researchers to a decreased risk of cognitive decline.

The recipes in this chapter prove that there is more to poultry than the default "health food" meal of chicken breast, rice, and broccoli. Once you try Chicken Chile Verde (page 119) and Coq au Vin (page 121), for instance, you'll discover a new excitement for these lean proteins—and you'll have no problem meeting the weekly MIND diet requirement of two poultry servings per week.

FRESH FOODS

A 2017 study published in the *Journal of the American Medical Association* found that nearly 50 percent of deaths from heart disease, stroke, and type 2 diabetes (also known as cardiometabolic deaths) in the United States are associated with a diet consisting of too much salt and processed meats, and not enough nuts/seeds and omega-3 fats. MIND diet researchers have shown that a diet rich in fresh produce and meats—including poultry—can help reduce the risk of cardiovascular-related diseases like hypertension, diabetes, heart attacks, and strokes. In addition to the poultry itself, which has its own health benefits, the recipes in this chapter also include a rainbow of fresh vegetables and other ingredients that liven up your plate without the need for excess salt, fat, and other unbeneficial ingredients.

See turkey in a new light with Turkey Tacos (page 129), Turkey Burgers (page 126), Turkey Meatballs (page 128), Turkey-Cranberry Rice (page 127), and Turkey with Barley and Squash (page 130). Use chicken breast in new ways with Artichoke Chicken (page 116), Asian-Inspired Chicken Rice Bowl (page 115), Mexican-Inspired Chicken Rice Bowl (page 124), Bok Choy and Chicken Stir-Fry (page 118), Chicken Lo Mein (page 120), and Grilled Chicken with Radish Relish (page 123).

ASIAN-INSPIRED CHICKEN RICE BOWL

30 MINUTES

SERVES 4 / PREP TIME: 10 MINUTES / COOK TIME: 20 MINUTES

Asian take-out food is an American favorite, from egg rolls to sesame chicken, and fried rice to fried meats in sweet-and-sour sauce. This recipe is an example of learning to make MIND diet–friendly versions of take-out favorites. Rice bowls are popular at many chains and can easily be made healthier at home.

2 cups water

1 cup brown rice

2 tablespoons olive oil

1 tablespoon minced garlic

1 red bell pepper, cut into strips

1 cup shelled edamame

1 cup cremini mushrooms, sliced

1 pound boneless, skinless chicken breasts, cubed

FOR THE TERIYAKI SAUCE

2 tablespoons low-sodium soy sauce

½ cup water

1 tablespoon honey

1 teaspoon ground ginger

1. In a large pot, bring the water to a boil.

2. Add the rice to the boiling water, reduce the heat to low, and cover. Cook for 15 to 20 minutes, until all the water is absorbed.

3. While the rice is cooking, in a large sauté pan or skillet, heat the olive oil over medium-high heat until shimmering.

4. Sauté the garlic, bell pepper, edamame, and mushrooms for 5 minutes.

5. Add the cubed chicken and cook for 5 to 7 minutes, until the chicken is cooked through.

6. While the chicken is cooking, in a small bowl, make the teriyaki sauce by whisking together the soy sauce, water, honey, and ginger.

7. Serve each bowl of rice, chicken, and vegetables topped with the teriyaki sauce.

SUBSTITUTION TIP: Make this recipe gluten-free by substituting tamari for the soy sauce.

PER SERVING: Calories: 419; Total fat: 12g; Protein: 34g; Carbohydrates: 48g; Fiber: 3g; Sugar: 6g; Sodium: 504mg

ARTICHOKE CHICKEN

GLUTEN-FREE
SERVES 2 TO 4 / PREP TIME: 20 MINUTES / COOK TIME: 30 MINUTES

Artichokes are a Mediterranean thistle high in vitamins C and K, folate, magnesium, and potassium. They are one of the vegetables highest in antioxidants as well as being full of fiber and plant-based protein. Artichokes have also been found to improve cholesterol levels, which is a cardiovascular benefit on the MIND diet.

4 artichokes

2 cups water

2 tablespoons lemon juice

2 tablespoons olive oil

1 pound boneless, skinless chicken breasts

½ cup low-sodium chicken stock

2 cups baby spinach

½ cup sun-dried tomatoes

1 teaspoon dried rosemary

1 teaspoon dried oregano

½ teaspoon freshly ground black pepper

1. On a cutting board, using a sharp serrated knife, cut off the top third of the artichokes, as this portion is inedible. Also cut off the bottom half of the stems.

2. Peel back the leaves until the yellow center is exposed. Using a small knife, cut away any woody bits near the base of the artichoke. Use a spoon or melon baller to remove the fibrous center of the artichoke heart.

3. In a large pot, cover the artichoke hearts with water and add the lemon juice. Cover with a lid and bring the water to a boil over medium-high heat. Cook for 20 minutes. Drain and set the artichokes aside.

4. While the artichokes are cooking, in a large and deep sauté pan or skillet, heat the olive oil on medium heat until shimmering.

5. Add the chicken breasts and cook each side for 5 to 7 minutes, or until the internal temperature reaches 165°F.

6. When the chicken is cooked through, dice the artichoke hearts and add to the pan.

7. Add the chicken stock, spinach, tomatoes, rosemary, oregano, and pepper. Cover the pan and cook for 5 minutes.

8. Serve each chicken breast on a bed of the vegetables with a drizzle of the pan sauce on top.

COOKING TIP: To cut down on food waste, you can prepare the artichokes using the same method as used in Sardines with Artichokes and Greens (page 104) and reserve the tender leaves for a snack.

PER SERVING: Calories: 513; Total fat: 20g; Protein: 58g; Carbohydrates: 38g; Fiber: 17g; Sugar: 8g; Sodium: 928mg

BOK CHOY AND CHICKEN STIR-FRY

GLUTEN-FREE, 30 MINUTES
SERVES 4 / PREP TIME: 10 MINUTES / COOK TIME: 20 MINUTES

Bok choy contains a high amount of antioxidants and anti-inflammatory nutrients in the form of selenium, vitamins C and E, and beta carotene. Incorporating bok choy into the MIND diet helps protect the brain from free radicals. This cruciferous vegetable is delicious in stir-fry and provides a serving of leafy green vegetables to your diet. Serve over your favorite noodles or rice.

2 tablespoons olive oil

2 tablespoons minced garlic

2 carrots, sliced

1 large head bok choy, coarsely chopped

1 pound boneless, skinless chicken breasts, cubed

1 tablespoon honey

2 tablespoons white wine vinegar

½ teaspoon ground ginger

½ teaspoon cayenne pepper

1. In a large sauté pan or skillet, heat the olive oil over medium-high heat until shimmering.

2. Sauté the garlic, carrots, and bok choy for 5 minutes.

3. Add the chicken and cook for 5 to 7 minutes, until the chicken is cooked through.

4. While the chicken is cooking, in a small bowl, whisk together the honey, vinegar, ginger, and cayenne pepper.

5. Add the sauce to the pan and stir-fry for 5 minutes. Serve.

SUBSTITUTION TIP: Make this recipe vegan by using Scrambled Tofu (page 22) instead of chicken.

PER SERVING: Calories: 215; Total fat: 10g; Protein: 25g; Carbohydrates: 10g; Fiber: 1g; Sugar: 6g; Sodium: 237mg

CHICKEN CHILE VERDE

GLUTEN-FREE, ONE-POT, SLOW COOKER

SERVES 4 / PREP TIME: 10 MINUTES / COOK TIME: 8 HOURS

Green chiles are a regional staple in the Southwest that add a tangy and crisp flavor without packing too much heat. They are rich in vitamins A, B_6, C, and K as well as potassium and copper. Chile peppers are also good sources of carotenoids, sinapic acid, and ferulic acid, all powerful antioxidants perfect for the MIND diet.

1 pound boneless, skinless chicken thighs

1 (27-ounce) can whole green chiles, drained and diced

1 yellow onion, diced

2 cups low-sodium chicken stock

2 tablespoons minced garlic

1 teaspoon ground cumin

1 teaspoon smoked paprika

2 tablespoons dried oregano

1 large avocado, pitted, peeled, and sliced

1. In a slow cooker, combine the chicken thighs, green chiles, onion, chicken stock, garlic, cumin, paprika, and oregano.

2. Cover and cook on low for 8 hours.

3. Serve each chicken thigh with a spoonful of the green chile sauce, topped with avocado slices.

INGREDIENT TIP: If you can find roasted Hatch green chiles where you live, they are a wonderful treat and add a roasted flavor to this dish.

COOKING TIP: You can cook this recipe on high for 4 hours, or on low for 8 hours.

PER SERVING: Calories: 275; Total fat: 15g; Protein: 20g; Carbohydrates: 18g; Fiber: 7g; Sugar: 6g; Sodium: 240mg

CHICKEN LO MEIN

30 MINUTES

SERVES 4 / PREP TIME: 15 MINUTES / COOK TIME: 15 MINUTES

Lo mein is a traditional Chinese dish made with egg noodles, vegetables, and often a meat protein. It has gained popularity in America and is stir-fried in a thin sauce made with soy sauce. This variation uses whole-grain spaghetti in place of the egg noodles to satisfy a MIND diet serving of whole grains and is full of vegetables. Stir-fry is often high in sodium, but this recipe has less sodium because it uses low-sodium ingredients like chicken stock and soy sauce in small amounts.

4 cups water

4 ounces whole-grain spaghetti

2 tablespoons olive oil

1 tablespoon minced garlic

1 orange bell pepper, cut into strips

1 broccoli crown, chopped

2 carrots, thinly sliced

1 pound boneless, skinless chicken breasts, cubed

1 cup low-sodium chicken stock

2 tablespoons low-sodium soy sauce

1 teaspoon ground ginger

Red pepper flakes

1. In a large pot, bring the water to a boil.

2. Boil the pasta for 10 to 12 minutes, until tender. Drain.

3. In a large and deep sauté pan or skillet, heat the olive oil over medium-high heat until shimmering.

4. Sauté the garlic, bell pepper, broccoli, and carrots for 5 minutes.

5. Add the cubed chicken and cook for 5 to 7 minutes, until cooked through.

6. Add the cooked pasta, chicken stock, soy sauce, and ginger and simmer for 5 minutes.

7. Serve with a sprinkling of red pepper flakes.

SUBSTITUTION TIP: Make this recipe gluten-free by substituting your favorite gluten-free noodles and tamari for the soy sauce.

PER SERVING: Calories: 317; Total fat: 11g; Protein: 29g; Carbohydrates: 29g; Fiber: 5g; Sugar: 4g; Sodium: 534mg

COQ AU VIN

GLUTEN-FREE, ONE-POT, SLOW COOKER
SERVES 4 / PREP TIME: 10 MINUTES / COOK TIME: 8 HOURS

Coq au vin is a classic French dish of chicken stewed in wine with vegetables, translated as "rooster with wine." This rustic preparation was used to make tougher cuts of poultry tender. Cooking with red wine is an excellent way to incorporate antioxidants into your diet.

1 pound boneless, skinless chicken thighs

1 (750 ml) bottle red burgundy wine

2 cups low-sodium chicken stock

1 tablespoon no-salt-added tomato paste

1 pound carrots, thinly sliced

1 leek, thinly sliced

½ pound cremini mushrooms

½ pound pearl onions, peeled

2 tablespoons minced garlic

1 teaspoon dried thyme

1. In a slow cooker, combine all the ingredients.

2. Cover and cook on low for 8 hours.

3. Serve each chicken thigh with a spoonful of stewed vegetables and a drizzle of the wine sauce.

INGREDIENT TIP: Choose a red burgundy wine that you would enjoy drinking, but not a bottle that would break the bank.

COOKING TIP: You can also cook this recipe on high for 4 hours.

PER SERVING: Calories: 409; Total fat: 7g; Protein: 22g; Carbohydrates: 32g; Fiber: 4g; Sugar: 11g; Sodium: 333mg

ESCAROLE-LEEK CHICKEN

GLUTEN-FREE, 30 MINUTES
SERVES 4 / PREP TIME: 10 MINUTES / COOK TIME: 15 MINUTES

Escarole is a bitter lettuce rich in calcium, iron, selenium, vitamin A, B vitamins, and vitamin C. A good source of beta carotene, escarole has important antioxidants that fight free radicals in the body. Leeks are a mild-flavored vegetable related to scallions, chives, shallots, onions, and garlic, all of which work to reduce inflammation. They are high in vitamin A carotenoids, vitamin C, manganese, and vitamin K.

2 tablespoons olive oil

3 tablespoons minced garlic

1 pound boneless, skinless chicken thighs

1 head escarole, sliced into ribbons

1 leek, thinly sliced

1 teaspoon dried thyme

¼ teaspoon red pepper flakes

1. In a large and deep sauté pan or skillet, heat the olive oil over medium-high heat until shimmering. Add the garlic and cook until fragrant, about 1 minute.

2. Sear the chicken thighs and cook for 5 minutes, flip over, and sear the other side and cook for 5 minutes.

3. Add the escarole, leek, thyme, and red pepper flakes.

4. Cover the pan and let the vegetables wilt for 5 minutes.

5. Serve each chicken thigh on a bed of sautéed escarole and leeks.

COOKING TIP: You can also make this recipe in the oven by roasting the ingredients on a baking sheet covered with aluminum foil.

PER SERVING: Calories: 246; Total fat: 14g; Protein: 19g; Carbohydrates: 12g; Fiber: 5g; Sugar: 2g; Sodium: 198mg

GRILLED CHICKEN WITH RADISH RELISH

GLUTEN-FREE, 30 MINUTES
SERVES 4 / PREP TIME: 15 MINUTES / COOK TIME: 15 MINUTES

Radishes are root vegetables with a sharp, spicy, peppery flavor. They are high in the antioxidant anthocyanin, which gives them their deep color. They are also high in vitamins A, B6, C, E, and K, boosting their antioxidant and anti-inflammatory properties. They are also a good source of potassium.

1 pound boneless, skinless chicken breasts

2 tablespoons olive oil

Freshly ground black pepper

1 bunch red radishes, finely sliced

1 cucumber, finely sliced

½ red onion, finely sliced

1 tablespoon white wine vinegar

1 tablespoon lime juice

½ teaspoon ground cumin

1. Preheat the grill on medium-high heat.

2. Brush the chicken breasts with the olive oil and season with black pepper.

3. Grill the chicken for 5 to 7 minutes, flip, and grill the other side for 5 to 7 minutes, until cooked through and a thermometer reads 165°F.

4. While the chicken is grilling, in a medium bowl, combine the radishes, cucumber, onion, vinegar, lime juice, and cumin. Set aside.

5. Serve each chicken breast topped with the radish relish.

COOKING TIP: You can also grill the chicken on a stovetop grill pan.

PER SERVING: Calories: 189; Total fat: 10g; Protein: 24g; Carbohydrates: 4g; Fiber: 1g; Sugar: 2g; Sodium: 185mg

MEXICAN-INSPIRED CHICKEN RICE BOWL

GLUTEN-FREE

SERVES 4 / PREP TIME: 15 MINUTES / COOK TIME: 20 MINUTES

Chicken and rice burritos and burrito bowls are the top sellers at Mexican fast-casual chains. The most popular of these chains has thousands of locations nationwide. The problem is that these tasty bowls are loaded with sodium and often topped with piles of cheese and gobs of sour cream. These Mexican-inspired chicken rice bowls are completely MIND diet–friendly and still pack a ton of flavor and are very low in sodium.

2 cups water

1 cup brown rice

2 tablespoons olive oil

1 tablespoon minced garlic

1 pound boneless, skinless chicken breasts, cubed

1 (15-ounce) can no-salt-added black beans, drained and rinsed

½ cup low-sodium chicken stock

1 teaspoon ground cumin

1 teaspoon chili powder

1 teaspoon chipotle chile powder

1 teaspoon dried oregano

½ cup chopped fresh cilantro

½ cup diced red onion

1 lime, halved

1. In a large pot, bring the water to a boil.

2. Add the rice to the boiling water, reduce the heat to low, and cover. Cook for 15 to 20 minutes, until all the water is absorbed.

3. While the rice is cooking, in a large sauté pan or skillet, heat the olive oil over medium heat until shimmering. Add the garlic and cook until fragrant, about 1 minute.

4. Add the chicken, beans, chicken stock, cumin, chili powder, chipotle chile powder, and oregano and cook, stirring, for 10 to 12 minutes.

5. Serve each bowl of rice, chicken, and beans topped with a sprinkle of cilantro, red onion, and a squeeze of fresh lime juice.

INGREDIENT TIP: The guacamole and salsa from chapter 3 (page 30) would go perfectly on these rice bowls.

PER SERVING: Calories: 452; Total fat: 12g; Protein: 34g; Carbohydrates: 58g; Fiber: 9g; Sugar: 2g; Sodium: 221mg

PARSLEY-STUFFED GAME HENS WITH ROASTED VEGETABLES

GLUTEN-FREE, ONE-POT

SERVES 2 TO 4 / PREP TIME: 15 MINUTES / COOK TIME: 1 HOUR 20 MINUTES

Game hens are actually not game birds at all. They are domestically raised for meat and have a large breast compared to their small size. Cooking with game hens is a fun way for each person to have their own little chicken and you get to enjoy both white meat and dark meat from the breast, thighs, and legs. The wings have very little meat to offer, but a game hen provides plenty of meat for one person or two people to share. This recipe is a good example of how eating healthy poultry does not always have to mean chicken breast!

2 Cornish game hens, without giblets

3 tablespoons olive oil, divided

1 teaspoon freshly ground black pepper, divided

1 bunch parsley, finely chopped

1 yam or sweet potato, scrubbed and diced

1 turnip, peeled and diced

1 acorn squash, peeled, seeded, and diced

1 yellow onion, sliced

1. Preheat the oven to 375°F.

2. Pat the hens dry and rub each with 1 tablespoon of olive oil, then season each with ½ teaspoon of pepper.

3. Stuff each hen with half of the chopped parsley.

4. On a large foil-lined baking sheet, roast the hens for 40 minutes.

5. Remove the pan from the oven and add the yam, turnip, squash, and onion in a single layer around the hens. Drizzle with the remaining olive oil.

6. Roast the hens and the vegetables for 40 more minutes. The internal temperature of the breasts must reach 165°F.

7. Serve the game hens on a bed of the roasted vegetables.

COOKING TIP: If you have an air fryer, these game hens can be cooked rotisserie style.

PER SERVING: Calories: 1,112; Total fat: 74g; Protein: 69g; Carbohydrates: 51g; Fiber: 9g; Sugar: 8g; Sodium: 314mg

TURKEY BURGERS

GLUTEN-FREE, ONE-POT
SERVES 4 / PREP TIME: 10 MINUTES / COOK TIME: 30 MINUTES

Turkey burgers are a great way to enjoy an American favorite and stay solid on the MIND diet. Ground turkey is moist and flavorful and takes on the delicious flavor of red bell pepper in this preparation. Turkey is a great source of the antioxidant mineral selenium, vitamin B6, zinc, and phosphorus.

1 pound ground turkey,
93% lean

1 red bell pepper, finely minced

**¼ cup gluten-free
bread crumbs**

¼ teaspoon garlic powder

¼ teaspoon onion powder

**4 gluten-free hamburger buns
or large iceberg lettuce leaves**

1 hothouse tomato, sliced

½ red onion, sliced

1. Preheat the grill on medium-high heat.

2. In a large bowl, combine the turkey, bell pepper, bread crumbs, garlic powder, and onion powder until all the ingredients are well incorporated.

3. Split the mixture into quarters and shape four patties.

4. Grill the patties for 5 to 7 minutes, flip, and grill the other side for 5 to 7 minutes, until cooked through and a thermometer reads 165°F.

5. Serve on a whole-grain bun or in a lettuce wrap, topped with the tomato and onion.

COOKING TIP: You can also grill the burgers on a stovetop grill pan.

PER SERVING: Calories: 392; Total fat: 13g; Protein: 28g; Carbohydrates: 43g; Fiber: 5g; Sugar: 6g; Sodium: 409mg

TURKEY-CRANBERRY RICE

GLUTEN-FREE, 30 MINUTES

SERVES 4 / PREP TIME: 10 MINUTES / COOK TIME: 20 MINUTES

Turkey is not just for Thanksgiving! It is a lean protein option on the MIND diet that is juicy and full of flavor, providing additional variety from chicken. Nutritionally, turkey and chicken are very similar, the only difference being that turkey is slightly higher in fat.

2 cups water

1 cup brown rice

1 cup fresh cranberries

1 pound boneless, skinless turkey breast, sliced

1 tablespoon dried rosemary

1 tablespoon dried sage

2 teaspoons dried thyme

2 tablespoons olive oil

Grated zest of 1 orange

1. In a large pot, bring the water to a boil.

2. Add the rice and cranberries to the boiling water, reduce the heat to low, and cover. Cook for 15 to 20 minutes, until all the water is absorbed.

3. While the rice and cranberries are cooking, rub the turkey breast with the rosemary, sage, and thyme.

4. In a large sauté pan or skillet, heat the olive oil over medium-high heat until shimmering.

5. Cook the turkey in a single layer for 5 to 7 minutes per side, until the internal temperature reaches 165°F.

6. Add the orange zest to the cranberry rice.

7. Serve each slice of turkey breast on a bed of the cranberry rice.

COOKING TIP: Because turkey breasts can be rather large, you can freeze the remaining turkey for future use.

PER SERVING: Calories: 363; Total fat: 11g; Protein: 28g; Carbohydrates: 43g; Fiber: 5g; Sugar: 4g; Sodium: 181mg

TURKEY MEATBALLS

GLUTEN-FREE

SERVES 4 / PREP TIME: 10 MINUTES / COOK TIME: 30 MINUTES

Parsley is not just a way to give food some green color. It is a delicious herb that packs a nutritious punch. It is very high in vitamin A and vitamin K, which are powerful antioxidants, and high in vitamin C. Parsley also has other antioxidants: flavonoids and carotenoids. Serve over whole-grain or gluten-free pasta, or in a hoagie roll for a meatball sub.

FOR THE MEATBALLS

1 pound ground turkey, 93% lean

1 bunch parsley, finely minced

¼ cup gluten-free bread crumbs

¼ teaspoon garlic powder

¼ teaspoon onion powder

2 tablespoons olive oil

FOR THE TOMATO SAUCE

1 (15-ounce) can no-salt-added tomato sauce

1 teaspoon garlic powder

1 teaspoon onion powder

1 tablespoon Italian seasoning

¼ cup low-sodium chicken stock

1. In a large bowl, mix the ground turkey, parsley, bread crumbs, garlic powder, and onion powder.

2. Roll the mixture into small meatballs, about 2 tablespoons in size. The turkey mixture should yield 20 meatballs.

3. In a large sauté pan or skillet, heat the olive oil on medium heat until the oil begins to shimmer.

4. Brown the meatballs for 2 minutes each side.

5. Add the tomato sauce, garlic powder, onion powder, and Italian seasoning and bring to low boil.

6. Add the chicken stock to deglaze the bottom of the pan.

7. Cook the meatballs in the sauce for 10 minutes, covered. Serve.

SUBSTITUTION TIP: If you do not have fresh parsley, dried parsley works just as well in this recipe, and retains its antioxidant properties. The conversion for fresh herbs to dried is 1:⅓. Use ⅓ cup dried parsley in this recipe.

PER SERVING: Calories: 287; Total fat: 15; Protein: 24g; Carbohydrates: 14g; Fiber: 4g; Sugar: 4g; Sodium: 156mg

TURKEY TACOS

GLUTEN-FREE, 30 MINUTES

SERVES 4 / PREP TIME: 10 MINUTES / COOK TIME: 20 MINUTES

By adding vegetables and beans to the turkey in these tacos, each serving is lower fat, lower calorie, higher fiber, and contains more nutrients than if it were made with meat alone. These tacos are more nutritious and healthier than restaurant or fast-food tacos. The moisture from the vegetables also keeps the turkey juicy with no added fat.

1 pound ground turkey, 93% lean

1 zucchini

1 carrot

1 (15-ounce) can no-salt-added pinto beans, drained and rinsed

1 (8-ounce) can no-salt-added tomato sauce

1 tablespoon dried oregano

1 teaspoon chili powder

1 teaspoon garlic powder

1 teaspoon onion powder

8 corn tortillas

1 cup mixed spring greens

1 small Roma tomato, diced

1. In a large sauté pan or skillet over medium heat, cook the turkey for 4 to 5 minutes, until no longer pink.

2. While the turkey is cooking, over a medium bowl, grate the zucchini and carrot.

3. Add the zucchini, carrot, beans, tomato sauce, oregano, chili powder, garlic powder, and onion powder to the browned turkey. Mix the ingredients together and cook for 15 minutes.

4. In a separate sauté pan or skillet, brown the corn tortillas on high heat in batches for 1 minute per side.

5. Build each taco with 2 to 3 tablespoons of the taco mixture. Top with spring greens and tomato. Serve.

SUBSTITUTION TIP: You can substitute crunchy corn taco shells for the soft corn tortillas.

INGREDIENT TIP: The guacamole and salsa from chapter 3 (page 30) would make a perfect addition to these simple but delicious tacos.

PER SERVING: Calories: 415; Total fat: 10g; Protein: 33g; Carbohydrates: 50g; Fiber: 11g; Sugar: 6g; Sodium: 162mg

TURKEY WITH BARLEY AND SQUASH

CONTAINS NUTS

SERVES 2 TO 4 / PREP TIME: 10 MINUTES / COOK TIME: 45 MINUTES

Yellow squash, also known as summer squash, is high in minerals and antioxidants. It is a good source of carotenoids, particularly beta-cryptoxanthin. This antioxidant is related to decreasing degenerative disease. Squash has a beautiful fresh flavor, enhanced by simple seasoning.

1½ cups low-sodium chicken stock

½ cup hulled barley

3 medium yellow squash

½ yellow onion

1 pound ground turkey, 93% lean

1 teaspoon freshly ground black pepper

¼ cup slivered almonds

1. In a medium pot, bring the chicken stock to a boil.

2. Add the barley to the boiling stock, reduce the heat to low, and cover. Cook for 40 minutes, until all the water is absorbed. (If the barley becomes dry before it has become chewy, add ½ cup water to the pan.)

3. While the barley is cooking, slice the squash and mince the onion.

4. In a large sauté pan or skillet over medium heat, cook the turkey for 4 to 5 minutes, or until no longer pink.

5. Add the squash, onion, and pepper to the browned turkey. Mix the ingredients together and cook for 15 minutes.

6. Serve the turkey and vegetables on a bed of barley with a sprinkling of slivered almonds.

INGREDIENT TIP: Hulled barley is a whole grain, as only the inedible hull has been removed. Pearl barley is the very center of the grain, a white starch that is not a whole grain. Pearl barley is what most people are familiar with in soups.

PER SERVING: Calories: 631; Total fat: 24g; Protein: 57g; Carbohydrates: 53g; Fiber: 12g; Sugar: 7g; Sodium: 303mg

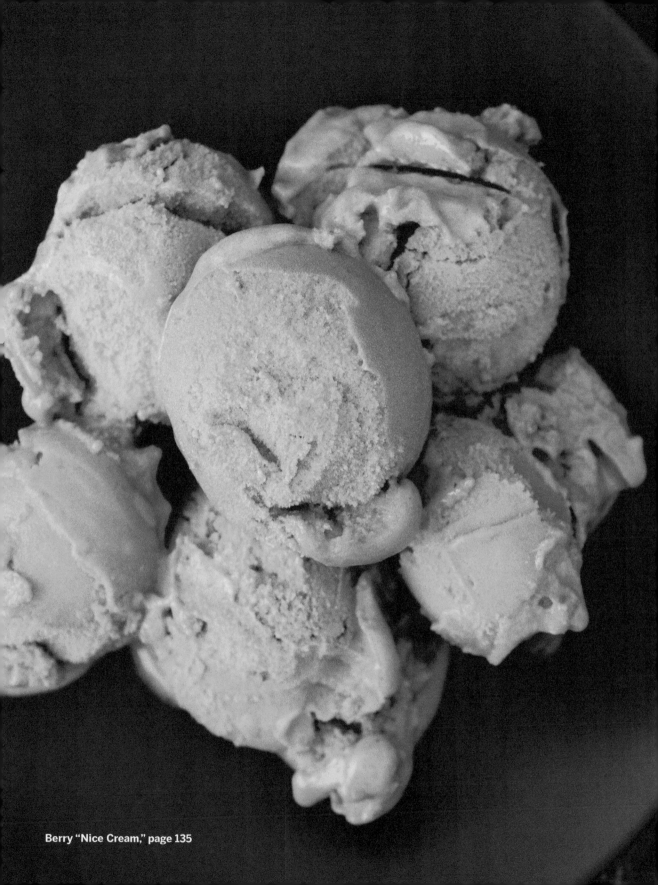

Berry "Nice Cream," page 135

DRINKS AND DESSERTS

On the MIND diet, desserts are welcome, as long as they are packed with antioxidants, vitamins, minerals, and fiber. The recipes in this chapter highlight the health benefits of delicious sweets like dark chocolate, red wine, and berries, and will help you find healthy ways to satisfy your sweet tooth while maintaining your MIND diet lifestyle.

Try MIND diet–friendly versions of dessert table favorites, such as Dark Chocolate and Date Brownies (page 139), Carrot Cupcakes (page 137), Berry Oat Crisp (page 136), Oatmeal Cookies and Coffee (page 143), Berry "Nice Cream" (page 135), and Dark Chocolate Bites (page 138). Sip refreshing antioxidant-packed drinks like Green Tea Soda (page 141), Green Juice (page 140), and Sangría (page 144), and see fruit in a new light with Grilled Watermelon and Pineapple (page 142). These recipes include minimal amounts of refined sugar, relying on the natural sweetness of dark chocolate, berries and other fruit, sweet vegetables, and wine.

Note: The recipes that follow are higher in sugar than those in the previous chapters, mostly due to ingredients like dark chocolate, fruit, and alcohol. Feel free to adapt these recipes to meet your specific health needs.

SUGAR

Sugar itself is not the enemy. Rather, health problems arise when refined sugar is consumed in excess. It is important to know the difference between naturally occurring sugars and refined sugar. Sugar is a natural nutrient contained in fruits, vegetables, and grains (in the forms of fructose, glucose, and sucrose), and in dairy (in the form of lactose). Refined sugar, on the other hand, is any sugar that is not found naturally in a whole food, such as sugar added to baked goods to improve the crumb quality and tenderness, sugar added to nondairy milks, sugar added to instant oatmeal packets, and the more obvious sweetened products like candy, cookies, ice cream, and beverages like sodas, flavored bottled teas, trendy coffee drinks, and energy drinks. Maintaining a diet low in refined sugar is important for achieving health and preventing chronic disease. Refined sugar is by no means off-limits on the MIND diet, but choosing naturally sweet whole foods is a better option for the health of your body and mind.

BERRY "NICE CREAM"

GLUTEN-FREE, ONE-POT, 30 MINUTES, VEGAN
SERVES 2 TO 4 / PREP TIME: 5 MINUTES

Ice cream is an American favorite, with the average American eating over 20 pounds of it per year. Typically made with heavy cream and sugar, ice cream is very high in calories per serving. This berry "nice cream" is equal in creaminess and sweetness without the added fat and sugar. This recipe is like fruit sorbet without the added sugar.

1 cup frozen strawberries

1 cup frozen raspberries

2 frozen bananas

1 tablespoon chopped fresh mint

1. In a blender, blend the frozen strawberries, raspberries, and bananas on high, or on the purée setting for 30 to 60 seconds.

2. Sprinkle each serving with fresh mint.

3. Serve immediately.

SUBSTITUTION TIP: Any blend of berries would work in this recipe.

PER SERVING: Calories: 167; Total fat: 1g; Protein: 3g; Carbohydrates: 42g; Fiber: 9g; Sugar: 21g; Sodium: 4mg

BERRY OAT CRISP

MAKES 9 SQUARES / PREP TIME: 10 MINUTES / COOK TIME: 40 MINUTES

Oats are a whole grain rich in plant-based protein, fiber, vitamins, minerals, and antioxidants. Incorporating oats into the MIND diet is an excellent way to meet your whole- grain requirements. Oats are extremely high in manganese, and a good source of B vitamins, phosphorus, magnesium, copper, iron, zinc, and folate. They contain high amounts of polyphenols and powerful antioxidants called avenanthramides.

2 cups blueberries, rinsed

2 cups raspberries, rinsed

2 cups blackberries, rinsed

1 tablespoon lemon juice

2 tablespoons cornstarch

¾ cup old-fashioned rolled oats

¼ cup whole-wheat flour

1 teaspoon ground cinnamon

¼ cup olive oil

¼ cup honey

1. Preheat the oven to 375°F.

2. In a medium bowl, combine the blueberries, raspberries, blackberries, lemon juice, and cornstarch. Mix well.

3. Fill a 9-by-9-inch baking dish with the berry mixture.

4. In a second medium bowl, combine the oats, flour, cinnamon, olive oil, and honey. Mix well.

5. Cover the berry mixture with the oat topping.

6. Bake for 35 to 40 minutes, or until the top has become golden brown and crisp.

7. Serve warm.

SUBSTITUTION TIP: Any blend of berries works well in this recipe.

PER SERVING: Calories: 174; Total fat: 7g; Protein: 2g; Carbohydrates: 28g; Fiber: 6g; Sugar: 14g; Sodium: 3mg

CARROT CUPCAKES

MAKES 12 CUPCAKES / PREP TIME: 15 MINUTES / COOK TIME: 25 MINUTES

Carrots are an excellent source of alpha and beta carotene. This antioxidant is important on the MIND diet, and adding surprise vegetables to these cupcakes makes dessert healthier. Carrots are also high in other antioxidants: lutein, lycopene, polyacetylenes and anthocyanins, vitamin A, vitamin B_6, vitamin K, potassium, and fiber.

Nonstick cooking spray

1 cup all-purpose flour

½ cup whole-wheat flour

1 teaspoon baking soda

1 teaspoon ground cinnamon

½ teaspoon ground ginger

½ cup pecan pieces

¼ cup olive oil

¼ cup unsweetened plain or vanilla nondairy milk

1 tablespoon white wine vinegar

¼ cup honey

1 (8-ounce) can crushed pineapple in 100% juice, undrained

2 medium carrots, scrubbed

Confectioners' sugar (optional)

1. Preheat the oven to 350°F. Coat a muffin tin with nonstick spray or use paper or silicone liners.

2. In a large bowl, combine the flours, baking soda, cinnamon, ginger, and pecans.

3. Add the olive oil, nondairy milk, vinegar, honey, and pineapple and its juice.

4. Mix until just combined.

5. Grate the carrots into the bowl and mix until just combined.

6. Fill each muffin cup with about 3 tablespoons of batter, or three-quarters full.

7. Bake for 20 to 25 minutes, or until the tops have browned and a toothpick inserted comes out clean.

8. Serve dusted with confectioners' sugar (if using).

SUBSTITUTION TIP: Make this recipe gluten-free by substituting your favorite gluten-free flour.

COOKING TIP: These cupcakes make a great grab-and-go breakfast.

PER SERVING: Calories: 163; Total fat: 8g; Protein: 2g; Carbohydrates: 22g; Fiber: 2g; Sugar: 9g; Sodium: 117mg

DARK CHOCOLATE BITES

CONTAINS NUTS, GLUTEN-FREE, VEGAN
MAKES 16 BITES / PREP TIME: 45 MINUTES

Dark chocolate is a decadent treat that is welcome on the MIND diet. Unlike milk chocolate, it has no milk solids and often much less added sugar. Dark chocolate is made from cacao solids, the beans from the cacao tree. The leftover powder from processing cacao beans is called cocoa powder. Per serving, dark chocolate is one of the best sources of antioxidants in the world, even more than açai berries and blueberries.

¾ cup old-fashioned rolled oats

¾ cup peanut butter or almond butter

¼ cup unsweetened cocoa powder

1 teaspoon vanilla extract

¼ cup vegan dark chocolate chips, 60% to 85% cacao

1. In a blender, purée the oats, nut butter, cocoa powder, and vanilla until a thick paste is made, about 30 seconds.

2. In a large bowl, combine the purée with the chocolate chips.

3. Make each bite using 2 tablespoons of the mixture. Roll into a ball and set on a plate.

4. Freeze the bites for 30 minutes.

5. Store in an airtight container in the refrigerator.

6. Serve whenever you need a sweet treat.

SUBSTITUTION TIP: Make this recipe nut-free by substituting sunflower seed butter for the peanut butter.

PER SERVING: Calories: 106; Total fat: 8g; Protein: 4g; Carbohydrates: 8g; Fiber: 2g; Sugar: 3g; Sodium: 57mg

DARK CHOCOLATE AND DATE BROWNIES

VEGAN

MAKES 9 SQUARES / PREP TIME: 15 MINUTES / COOK TIME: 25 MINUTES

Dates are the fruit from the date palm tree. They have a naturally high sugar content and make a great substitute for refined sugar. They have the added benefit of fiber, vitamins, minerals, and antioxidants, which regular sugar lacks. Dates contain flavonoids, carotenoids, and phenolic acid, antioxidants that work to reduce inflammation. Using dates as a sugar substitute is MIND diet friendly. Serve with a side of berries, if you like.

1 cup dates, pitted

½ cup hot water

1 cup all-purpose flour

¼ cup unsweetened cocoa powder

1 cup unsweetened plain or vanilla nondairy milk

⅓ cup olive oil

2 teaspoons vanilla extract

1 cup vegan dark chocolate chips, 60% to 85% cacao

1. Preheat the oven to 350°F.

2. In a blender, purée the dates and water until a thick paste is made, about 30 seconds.

3. In a large bowl, whisk together the flour and cocoa powder.

4. Add the nondairy milk, olive oil, and vanilla extract and mix well.

5. Add the date purée and chocolate chips to the mixture and mix well.

6. Fill a parchment paper–lined 9-by-9-inch baking dish with the batter.

7. Bake for 25 to 30 minutes, or until an inserted toothpick comes out clean.

8. Refrigerate the brownies for 1 to 2 hours before serving.

SUBSTITUTION TIP: Make this recipe gluten-free by substituting your favorite gluten-free flour.

PER SERVING: Calories: 306; Total fat: 17g; Protein: 2g; Carbohydrates: 42g; Fiber: 5g; Sugar: 25g; Sodium: 29mg

GREEN JUICE

GLUTEN-FREE, 30 MINUTES, VEGAN
SERVES 2 TO 4 / PREP TIME: 10 MINUTES

You don't need an expensive juicer for this recipe, or for any juicing recipe. You can make juice by blending fruit in a blender and then using a strainer to separate the juice from the pulp. The vibrant green ingredients in this recipe provide the gorgeous color of this juice, but the health impact is far more important. The antioxidants are ready to drink up!

2 Granny Smith apples, cored

2 cups spinach, packed

2 cucumbers

4 celery stalks

2 bunches parsley

2 cups water

1. In a blender, blend all the ingredients on high, or on the smoothie setting for 30 to 60 seconds.

2. Over a large bowl, strain the juice using cheesecloth or a fine-mesh strainer. Squeeze as much juice as you can out of the pulp by tightly wringing the cheesecloth or by repeatedly mashing the pulp into the strainer.

3. Discard the pulp and serve the reserved juice.

VARIATION TIP: To receive the added benefit of the fiber from these fruits and vegetables, make this recipe as a smoothie by adding a cup of ice instead of straining the juice from the mixture.

PER SERVING: Calories: 174; Total fat: 2g; Protein: 7g; Carbohydrates: 39g; Fiber: 12g; Sugar: 22g; Sodium: 167mg

GREEN TEA SODA

GLUTEN-FREE, 30 MINUTES, VEGAN
SERVES 8 / PREP TIME: 10 MINUTES

Green tea is a MIND diet superstar, packed with antioxidants. Sweetened beverages account for a large portion of excess calories and added sugar in the American diet. Replacing soda with sparkling water is a great alternative. Sparkling water and seltzer water do not contain any sweeteners or sodium, whereas club soda contains sodium and tonic water contains sodium and sugar.

2 cups water

4 green tea bags

2 cups ice

2 (12-ounce) cans sparkling water

1. In a large microwave-safe container, heat the water and the tea bags on high for 3 minutes.

2. Allow the tea to steep for 5 minutes, then remove the tea bags.

3. Fill a large pitcher with the ice.

4. Pour the hot tea over the ice and add the sparkling water. Stir together.

5. Serve chilled.

VARIATION TIP: Add fresh berries, citrus slices, or fresh mint to your green tea soda for a refreshing twist.

PER SERVING: Calories: 0; Total fat: 0g; Protein: 0g; Carbohydrates: 0g; Fiber: 0g; Sugar: 0g; Sodium: 0mg

GRILLED WATERMELON AND PINEAPPLE

GLUTEN-FREE, 30 MINUTES, VEGAN
SERVES 2 TO 4 / PREP TIME: 15 MINUTES / COOK TIME: 10 MINUTES

Watermelon has a very high water content, making it a refreshing fruit dessert. It is high in vitamins A and C as well as antioxidants like carotenoids, lycopene, and cucurbitacin E. Pineapple is high in vitamin C and manganese and contains powerful antioxidants like flavonoids and phenolic acid. This simple dessert works to fight free radicals and inflammation.

1 icebox watermelon

1 pineapple

Olive oil

1 lime, halved

1. Preheat the grill on high.

2. While the grill is heating up, cut the watermelon in half, then cut each half into 1-inch slices.

3. Peel and core the pineapple and cut into 1-inch rings or half-moon slices.

4. Brush the grill grate with olive oil.

5. Grill the watermelon and pineapple for 3 minutes per side.

6. Serve with a squeeze of fresh lime juice.

COOKING TIP: You can also grill the fruit on a stove-top grill pan.

PER SERVING: Calories: 217; Total fat: 2g; Protein: 3g; Carbohydrates: 56g; Fiber: 5g; Sugar: 43g; Sodium: 7mg

OATMEAL COOKIES AND COFFEE

VEGAN

MAKES 12 COOKIES / PREP TIME: 15 MINUTES / COOK TIME: 20 MINUTES

Coffee is MIND diet–friendly due to its strong antioxidant properties. It contains polyphenols, tannic acid, and caffeic acid, all powerful antioxidants. Coffee has been widely studied for brain health and helps prevent or delay cognitive decline.

½ cup whole-wheat flour

¼ cup sugar

½ teaspoon baking soda

1 teaspoon ground cinnamon

1 cup old-fashioned rolled oats

¼ cup olive oil

¼ cup plus 1 tablespoon unsweetened applesauce

1 teaspoon vanilla extract

1 cup brewed coffee per person

1. Preheat the oven to 375°F.

2. In a large bowl, whisk together the flour, sugar, baking soda, and cinnamon.

3. Add the oats, olive oil, applesauce, and vanilla and mix well.

4. Make each cookie from 2 tablespoons of batter, rolling into a ball, and then lightly pressing flat onto a parchment paper-lined baking sheet.

5. Bake for 10 minutes, or until the cookies have become golden brown.

6. Allow the cookies to rest on the baking sheet for 5 to 10 minutes to firm up as they cool.

7. Serve with a hot cup of coffee.

VARIATION TIP: Add ¼ cup raisins, dried cranberries, or dark chocolate chips to these cookies to add an antioxidant punch.

SUBSTITUTION TIP: If coffee is not to your taste, enjoy your cookies with a cup of tea.

PER SERVING: Calories: 102; Total fat: 5g; Protein: 2g; Carbohydrates: 13g; Fiber: 2g; Sugar: 5g; Sodium: 53mg

SANGRÍA

GLUTEN-FREE, VEGAN
SERVES 2 TO 4 / PREP TIME: 2 HOURS

Sangría is a Spanish beverage made from wine and fruit. It works well with both dry wines and sweet wines and can be made with red or white wine and any fruits. The MIND diet recommends 1 glass of red wine per day for the powerful antioxidant benefits. Red wine is a rich source of carotenoids, flavonoids, and polyphenols. If you prefer not to drink alcohol, 100% grape juice and 100% cranberry juice also contain high levels of antioxidants and are great substitutions for the wine.

2 cups blackberries, rinsed

2 oranges, sliced

1 lemon, sliced

1 (750mL) bottle red wine

1. In a large pitcher, mash half of the blackberries, orange slices, and lemon slices with a wooden spoon.

2. Add the wine and the remaining blackberries, orange slices, and lemon slices.

3. Refrigerate the mixture for at least 2 hours.

4. Serve over ice.

VARIATION TIP: Make nonalcoholic sangría by replacing the wine with 2 cups 100% grape juice or 100% cranberry juice, 1 tablespoon white wine vinegar, and 1 cup water.

PER SERVING: Calories: 465; Total fat: 1g; Protein: 3g; Carbohydrates: 49g; Fiber: 13g; Sugar: 22g; Sodium: 14mg

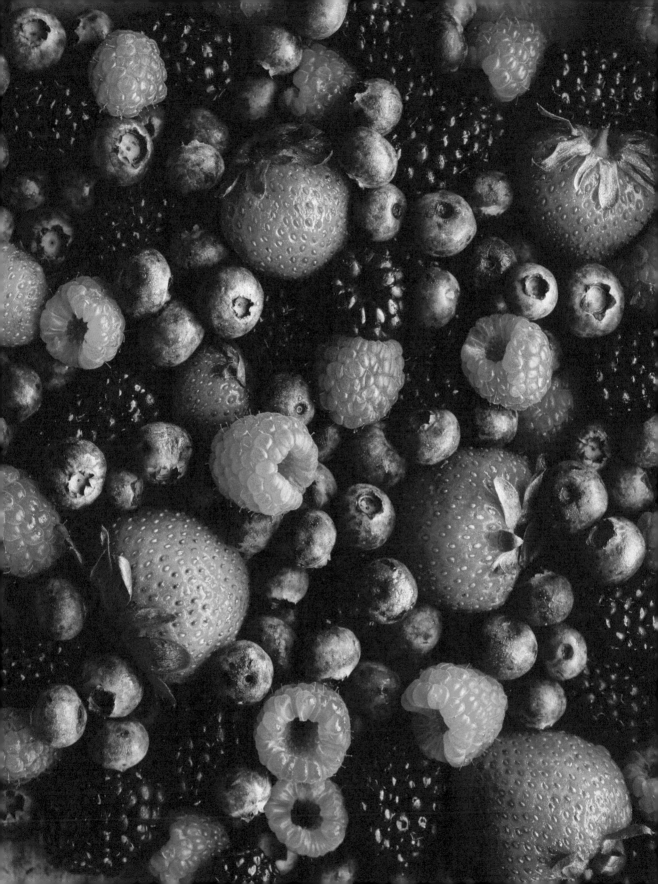

MEAL PLANS

Following the nutritional guidelines we listed for you on pp. 6 and 7, we have created this chart to help you keep track of MIND diet foods in every meal.

DAILY RECOMMENDATIONS:

- 3 servings of whole grains
- 1 salad with leafy greens
- 1 additional serving of vegetables
- 1 glass of red wine (optional)

WEEKLY RECOMMENDATIONS:

- Snack on nuts most days
- Eat ½ cup beans or other legumes 3 to 4 times per week
- Have poultry at least 2 times per week
- Eat ½ cup berries at least 2 times per week
- Have fish at least once per week
- Use olive oil for cooking and home-made salad dressings and marinades

	BREAKFAST	LUNCH	DINNER	SNACKS & DESSERT
EXAMPLE	Vegetable-Avocado Toast (1 serving whole grain, 1 serving vegetables)	Kale Succotash Salad (1 salad with leafy greens, 1 serving vegetables)	White Bean and Chicken Chili (poultry twice per week, beans 3 to 4 times per week)	Spicy Nut Mix Berries (snack on nuts most days, berries twice per week)
MONDAY				
TUESDAY				
WEDNESDAY				
THURSDAY				
FRIDAY				
SATURDAY				
SUNDAY				

MEASUREMENT CONVERSIONS

VOLUME EQUIVALENTS (LIQUID)

US STANDARD	US STANDARD (OUNCES)	METRIC (APPROXIMATE)
2 tablespoons	1 fl. oz.	30 mL
¼ cup	2 fl. oz.	60 mL
½ cup	4 fl. oz.	120 mL
1 cup	8 fl. oz.	240 mL
1½ cups	12 fl. oz.	355 mL
2 cups or 1 pint	16 fl. oz.	475 mL
4 cups or 1 quart	32 fl. oz.	1 L
1 gallon	128 fl. oz.	4 L

OVEN TEMPERATURES

FAHRENHEIT	CELSIUS (APPROXIMATE)
250°F	120°C
300°F	150°C
325°F	165°C
350°F	180°C
375°F	190°C
400°F	200°C
425°F	220°C
450°F	230°C

VOLUME EQUIVALENTS (DRY)

US STANDARD	METRIC (APPROXIMATE)
⅛ teaspoon	0.5 mL
¼ teaspoon	1 mL
½ teaspoon	2 mL
¾ teaspoon	4 mL
1 teaspoon	5 mL
1 tablespoon	15 mL
¼ cup	59 mL
⅓ cup	79 mL
½ cup	118 mL
⅔ cup	156 mL
¾ cup	177 mL
1 cup	235 mL
2 cups or 1 pint	475 mL
3 cups	700 mL
4 cups or 1 quart	1 L

WEIGHT EQUIVALENTS

US STANDARD	METRIC (APPROXIMATE)
½ ounce	15 g
1 ounce	30 g
2 ounces	60 g
4 ounces	115 g
8 ounces	225 g
12 ounces	340 g
16 ounces or 1 pound	455 g

REFERENCES

Barnes, Jennifer L., Min Tian, Neile K. Edens, and Martha Clare Morris. "Consideration of Nutrient Levels in Studies of Cognitive Decline: A Review." *Nutrition Reviews* 72, no. 11 (November 2014): 707-19. doi:10.1111/nure.12144.

Bennett, David A., Julie A. Schneider, Aron S. Buchman, Lisa L. Barnes, Patricia A. Boyle, and Robert S. Wilson. "Overview and Findings from the Rush Memory and Aging Project." *Current Alzheimer Research* 9, no. 6 (2012): 646–63. doi:10.2174/156720512801322663.

Calon, Frederic, Giselle P. Lim, Fusheng Yang, Takashi Morihara, Bruce Teter, Oliver Ubeda, Phillippe Rostaing, Antoine Triller, Norman Salem Jr., Karen H. Ashe, Sally A. Frautschy, and Greg M. Cole. "Docosahexaenoic Acid Protects from Dendritic Pathology in an Alzheimer's Disease Mouse Model." *Neuron* 43, no. 5 (September 2004): 633–45. doi:10.1016/j.neuron.2004.08.013.

Chen, X., Y. Huang, and H. Cheng. "Lower Intake of Vegetables and Legumes Associated with Cognitive Decline among Illiterate Elderly Chinese: A 3-Year Cohort Study." *Journal of Nutrition, Health & Aging* 16 (February 2012): 549–52. doi:10.1007/s12603-012-0023-2.

Devore, Elizabeth E., Jae Hee Kang, Monique M. B. Breteler, and Francine Grodstein. "Dietary Intakes of Berries and Flavonoids in Relation to Cognitive Decline." *Annals of Neurology* 72, no. 1 (April 2012): 135–43. doi:10.1002/ana.23594.

Ellingsworth, Christy, and Murdoc Khaleghi. *The Everything Guide to the MIND Diet*. Avon: Adams Media, 2016.

Feart, Catherine, Cecilia Samieri, and Virginie Rondeau. "Adherence to a Mediterranean Diet, Cognitive Decline, and Risk of Dementia" *Journal of the American Medical Association* 302, no. 22 (August 2009): 638–48. doi:10.1001/jama.2009.1146.

Guthrie, Joanne, and Biing-Hwan Lin. "Healthy Vegetables Undermined by the Company They Keep." United States Department of Agriculture Economic

Research Service (May 2014). www.ers.usda.gov/amber-waves/2014/may/healthy-vegetables-undermined-by-the-company-they-keep.

Joseph, J., N. A. Denisova, and G. Arendash. "Blueberry Supplementation Enhances Signaling and Prevents Behavioral Deficits in an Alzheimer Disease Model." *Nutritional Neuroscience* 6, no. 3 (2003): 153-62. doi:10.1080/1028415031000111282.

Joseph, J., B. Shukitt-Hale, N. A. Denisova, D. Bielinksi, A. Martin, J. J. McEwen, and P. C. Bickford. "Reversals of Age-Related Declines in Neuronal Signal Transduction, Cognitive, and Motor Behavioral Deficits with Blueberry, Spinach, or Strawberry Dietary Supplementation." *Journal of Neuroscience* 19, no. 18 (September 1999): 8114–21.

Kalmijn, S., L. J. Launer, A. Ott, J. C. Witteman, A. Hofman, and M. M. Breteler. "Dietary Fat Intake and the Risk of Incident Dementia in the Rotterdam Study." *Annals of Neurology* 42, no. 5 (November 1997): 776–82.

Kang, J. H., A. Ascherio, and F. Grodstein. "Fruit and Vegetable Consumption and Cognitive Decline in Aging Women." *Annals of Neurology* 57, no. 5 (May 2005): 713–20.

Lim, G. P., F. Calon, T. Morihara, F. Yang, B. Teter, O. Ubeda, N. Salem, Jr., S. A. Frautschy, and G. M. Cole. "A Diet Enriched with the Omega-3 Fatty Acid Docosahexaenoic Acid Reduces Amyloid Burden in an Aged Alzheimer Mouse Model." *Journal of Neuroscience* 25, no. 12 (March 2005): 3032–40.

Marcason, Wendy. "What Are the Components to the MIND Diet?" *Journal of the Academy of Nutrition and Dietetics* 115, no. 10 (October 2015): 1744. doi:10.1016/j.jand.2015.08.002.

Martinez-Lapiscina, E. H., P. Clavero, E. Toledo, R. Estruch, J. Salas-Salvado, B. San Julian, A. Sanchez-Tainta, E. Ros, C. Valls-Pedret, and M. A. Martinez-Gonzalez. "Mediterranean Diet Improves Cognition: The PREDIMED-NAVARRA Randomised Trial." *Journal of Neurology, Neurosurgery, and Psychiatry* 84, no. 12 (December 2013): 1318–25.

Micha, Renata et al. "Association Between Dietary Factors and Mortality from Heart Disease, Stroke, and Type 2 Diabetes in the United States." *Journal of *the American Medical Association* 317, no. 9 (2017): 912–924. doi:10.1001/jama.2017.0947.

Morris, Martha, D. A. Evans, and J. L. Bienias. "Consumption of Fish and n-3 Fatty Acids and Risk of Incident Alzheimer Disease." *Archives of Neurology* 60 (2003): 940-6.

Morris, Martha, D. A. Evans, Christy C. Tangney, J. L. Bienias, and R. S. Wilson. "Fish Consumption and Cognitive Decline with Age in a Large Community Study." *Archives of Neurology* 62 (2005): 1849-53.

Morris, Martha, D. A. Evans, Christy C. Tangney, J. L. Bienias, and R. S. Wilson. "Associations of Vegetable and Fruit Consumption with Age-Related Cognitive Change." *Neurology* 64, no. 8 (October 2006): 1370-6.

Morris, Martha, Christy C. Tangney, Yamin Wang, Frank M. Sacks, Lisa L. Barnes, David A. Bennett, and Neelum T. Aggarwal. "MIND Diet Slows Cognitive Decline with Aging." *Alzheimer's & Dementia* 11, no. 9 (September 2015): 1015-22. doi:10.1016/j.jalz.2015.04.011.

Morris, Martha, Christy C. Tangney, Yamin Wang, Frank M. Sacks, David A. Bennett, and Neelum T. Aggarwal. "MIND Diet Associated with Reduced Incidence of Alzheimer's Disease." *Alzheimer's & Dementia* 11, no. 9 (September 2015): 1007-14. doi:10.1016/j.jalz.2014.11.009.

Morris, Martha, and Christy C. Tangney. "Dietary Fat Composition and Dementia Risk". *Neurobiology of Aging* (2014). doi:10.1016/j.neurobiolaging.2014.03.038.

Morris, Martha, Christy C. Tangney, and Yamin Wang. "MIND Diet Score More Predictive than DASH or Mediterranean Diet Scores." *Alzheimer's & Dementia* (2014): 1-8. doi:10.1016/j.jalz.2014.11.009.

Morris, Martha. "Nutritional Determinants of Cognitive Aging and Dementia." *Proceedings of Nutrition Society* 71 (2012): 1-13.

Morris, Martha. *Diet for the MIND: The Latest Science for What to Eat to Prevent Alzheimer's and Cognitive Decline*. New York: Hachette Book Group, 2017.

Nishida, Y., S. Ito, S. Ohtsuki. "Depletion of Vitamin E Increases Amyloid Beta Accumulation by Decreasing Its Clearances from Brain and Blood in a Mouse Model of Alzheimer Disease." *Journal of Biological Chemistry* 284, no. 48 (2009): 33400–8.

Nooyens, Astrid C. J., H. Bas Bueno-de-Mesquita, Martin P. J. van Boxtel, Boukje M. van Gelder, Hans Verhagen, and W. M. Monique Verschuren. "Fruit and Vegetable Intake and Cognitive Decline in Middle-Aged Men and Women: The Doetinchem Cohort Study." *British Journal of Nutrition* 106, no. 5 (September 2011): 752–61. doi:10.1017/S0007114511001024.

Obulesu, M., Muralidhara Rao Dowlathabad, and P. V. Bramhachari. "Carotenoids and Alzheimer's Disease: An Insight into Therapeutic Role of Retinoids in Animal Models." *Neurochemistry International* 59, no. 5 (October 2011): 535–41. doi:10.1016/j.neuint.2011.04.004.

Roberts, Rosebud O., Yonus E. Geda, James R. Cerhan, David S. Knopman, Ruth H. Cha, Teresa J. H. Christianson, V. Shane Pankratz, Robert J. Ivnik, Bradley F. Boeve, Helen M. O'Connor, and Ronald C. Petersen. "Vegetables, Unsaturated Fats, Moderate Alcohol Intake, and Mild Cognitive Impairment." *Dementia and Geriatric Cognitive Disorders* 29, no. 5 (June 2010): 413–23. doi:10.1159/000305099.

Rush University Medical Center. "Diet May Help Prevent Alzheimer's: MIND Diet Rich in Vegetables, Berries, Whole Grains, Nuts." March 16, 2015. www.rush.edu/news/diet-may-help-prevent-alzheimers.

Scarmeas, Nikolaos, Yaakov Stern, Ming-Xin Tang, Richard Mayeux, and Jose A. Luchsinger. "Mediterranean Diet and Risk for Alzheimer's Disease." *Annals of Neurology* 56, no. 6 (June 2006): 912–21. doi:10.1002/ama.20854.

Sebastian, Rhonda S., Cecilia Wilkinson Enns, and Joseph D. Goldman. "Snacking Patterns of U.S. Adults." *What We Eat in America, NHANES 2007-2008*. Food Surveys Research Group Dietary Data Brief No. 4 (June 2011). www.ars.usda.gov/ARSUserFiles/80400530/pdf/DBrief/4 _adult_snacking_0708.pdf.

Sebastian, Rhonda S., et al. "Salad Consumption in the U.S." *What We Eat in America, NHANES 2011–2014.* Food Surveys Research Group Dietary Data Brief No. 19 (February 2018). www.ars.usda.gov/ARSUserFiles/80400530 /pdf/DBrief/19_Salad_consumption_2011_2014.pdf.

Tangney, Christine C., Mary J. Kwasny, Hong Li, Robert S. Wilson, Denis A. Evans, and Martha C. Morris. "Adherence to a Mediterranean-Type Dietary Pattern and Cognitive Decline in a Community Population." *American Journal of Clinical Nutrition* 93, no. 3 (December 2011): 601–7. doi:10.3945 /ajcn.110.007369.

Tangney, Christy C., Hong Li, and Y. Wang. "Relation of DASH- and Mediterranean-Like Dietary Patterns on Cognitive Decline in Older Persons." *Neurology* 83, no. 16 (October 2014): 1410–6. doi:10.1212/wnl .0000000000000884.

Tangney, Christine C., Hong Li, L. L. Barnes, J. A. Schneider, D. A. Bennett, and Martha C. Morris. "Accordance to Dietary Approaches to Stop Hypertension (DASH) Is Associated with Slower Cognitive Decline." *Alzheimer's & Dementia* 9 (2013): 605–6.

Tsivgoulis, Georgios, Suzanne Judd, Abraham J. Letter, Andrei V. Alexandrov, George Howard, Fadi Nahab, Frederick W. Unverzagt, Claudia Moy, Virginia J. Howard, Brett Kissela, and Virginia G. Wadley. "Adherence to a Mediterranean Diet and Risk of Incident Cognitive Impairment." *Neurology* 80, no. 18 (April 2013): 1684–92. doi:10.1212/WNL.0b013e3182904f69.

U.S. Department of Health and Human Services and U.S. Department of Agriculture. *2015– 2020 Dietary Guidelines for Americans.* 8th Edition. December 2015. health.gov/our-work/food-and-nutrition/2015-2020-dietary -guidelines.

Van de Rest, O., A. A. Berendsen, A. Haveman-Niles, and L. C. deGroot. "Dietary Patterns, Cognitive Decline, and Dementia: A Systematic Review." *Advances in Nutrition* 6 (2015). 154–68.

Wengreen, Heidi, Ronald G. Munger, Adele Cutler, Anna Quach, Austin Bowles, Christopher Corcoran, JoAnn T. Tschanz, Maria C. Norton, and Kathleen A. Welsh-Bohmer. "Prospective Study of Dietary Approaches to Stop Hypertension and Mediterranean-Style Dietary Patterns and Age-Related Cognitive Change: The Cache County Study on Memory, Health and Aging." *American Journal of Clinical Nutrition* 98, no. 5 (November 2013): 1263–71. doi:10.3945/ajcn.112.051276.

Willis, Lauren, Barbara Shukitt-Hale, and James A. Joseph. "Recent Advances in Berry Supplementation and Age-Related Cognitive Decline." *Current Opinion in Clinical Nutrition and Metabolic Care* 12, no. 1 (January 2009): 91-4. doi:10.1097/MCO.0b013e32831b9c6e.

INDEX

ACKNOWLEDGMENTS

I first and foremost want to thank my husband, Alden, and my daughter, Alyssa—my favorite people in the world. Thank you for giving me unlimited motivation, encouragement, and hugs, and for taste testing all my recipes without complaint. You are my reasons why.

Thank you to my dad, Mark, for encouraging me to write a book since I was a child. Thank you to my mom, Nannette, for always being my cheerleader and proofreader. You both always knew I could do it.

Thank you to my classmate, colleague, and role model Tara, for showing me that this dream was possible.

Last, but certainly not least, thank you to the wonderful team at Callisto, for making my dream of writing a book a reality. It has been an absolute pleasure working with you all.

ABOUT THE AUTHOR

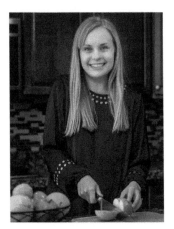

AMANDA FOOTE, RD, is a registered dietitian, proud fire wife, and mother. She runs her own virtual nutrition practice, Amanda Foote Nutrition, specializing in food allergies and intolerances, and special (therapeutic) diets for medical conditions that require following a specific diet. It is her calling to ensure that food remains an enjoyable, nourishing part of the human experience, despite dietary restrictions.

Amanda has worked as a registered dietitian for InnovAge and South Adams County Fire Department and is currently running her own nutrition practice. Amanda has a bachelor's degree in dietetics from the University of Northern Colorado and a bachelor's degree in applied psychology from Regis University.

Amanda lives in Colorado with her family and pets. In her spare time, she enjoys developing new recipes, sketching, crafting, reading, running 5Ks, and all things Disney.

CPSIA information can be obtained
at www.ICGtesting.com
Printed in the USA
BVHW091655310821
615706BV00012B/201

9 781646 117987